Titles previously published in
YOUR PERSONAL HEALTH SERIES

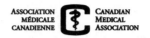

ASSOCIATION
MÉDICALE
CANADIENNE

CANADIAN
MEDICAL
ASSOCIATION

Parkinson's

Stepping Forward

David A. Grimes, MD

KEY PORTER BOOKS

National Library of Canada Cataloguing in Publication

Grimes, David A., 1966–
   Parkinson's stepping forward / David A. Grimes

(Your personal health series)
"Canadian Medical Association."
Includes bibliographical references and index.
ISBN 1-55263-266-0

1. Parkinson's disease—Popular works. I. Canadian Medical
Association. II. Title. III. Series.

RC382.G748 2004   616.8'33   C2003-905173-0

THE CANADA COUNCIL | LE CONSEIL DES ARTS
FOR THE ARTS | DU CANADA
SINCE 1957 | DEPUIS 1957

ONTARIO ARTS COUNCIL
CONSEIL DES ARTS DE L'ONTARIO

The publisher gratefully acknowledges the support of the Canada Council for the
Arts and the Ontario Arts Council for its publishing program.

We acknowledge the financial support of the Government of Canada through the
Book Publishing Industry Development Program (BPIDP) for our publishing activities.

We acknowledge the support of the Government of Ontario through the Ontario
Media Development Corporation's Ontario Book Initiative.

Key Porter Books Limited
70 The Esplanade
Toronto, Ontario
Canada M5E 1R2

www.keyporter.com

Design: Peter Maher
Electronic formatting: Heidy Lawrance Associates

Printed and bound in Canada

04 05 06 07 08 09 6 5 4 3 2 1

Contents

Acknowledgments

In life it is not only the obvious difficulties that matter, but small problems as well. For those with chronic illnesses it is often the seemingly minor things that really affect daily functioning; improving those may enable the person to retain dignity and independence. Compassion, encouragement and optimism are traits my father, J. David Grimes, embodied. This book is dedicated to him. He lived these qualities as a physician, and later as a patient. My father was a great believer in coping with illness and its limitations but then getting on with life. He was always Stepping Forward. He was an inspiration to his family, his friends, his colleagues and especially his patients. Thank you, Dad.

Thanks also to my wife, Joanne, whose daily encouragement, support and editing helped get this book written.

Foreword

D r. David Grimes, a senior Parkinson's disease expert, carries on a family tradition by adapting a book his father originally wrote, and bringing patients and caregivers a readable, educational resource about Parkinson's disease and its multiple dimensions. His message is a realistic and positive one, as he explains the disease and its elements and, at the same time, urges patients and families to take a proactive role in self-education, exercise, nutrition and other strategies to promote medical and social autonomy. Written with authoritative accuracy, yet in the style of a gentle family physician, this book will help any reader understand the challenges implicit in facing Parkinson's disease. Dr. Grimes explains typical problems related to tremor and bradykinesia, but also discusses less recognized impairments such as pain, sweating abnormalities, dental problems, and cognitive and emotional concerns. Other issues frequently raised by patients, such as the role of osteoporosis and estrogen replacement therapy, are explained with clarity, to the limits of our present scientific knowledge.

After the introductory material and the discussion of the physiological basis of Parkinson's disease, readers will likely be most interested in the chapter "Managing the Symptoms of Parkinson's," in which many practical suggestions, some general and some quite specific, are offered on a wide range of clinical problems. The general recommendations are solid strategies to maximize a patient's independence; the specific recommendations are useful and clearly explained, providing techniques for tackling a large number of common and not-so-common obstacles.

One point that cannot be overemphasized in the current context of new discoveries and new clinical trials is that people with Parkinson's disease and their families must never feel they are without choices. The number of new programs available at every phase of impairment is sufficiently large that the sense of desperation and lack of options that once accompanied this disease should no longer prevail. Though families and patients may need to travel to university centers or to consultants leading these new studies, there are now many options to empower them with choices.

Parkinson's: Stepping Forward offers several specific examples of new therapies, and each year, additional new discoveries are likely to expand patient opportunities. Beyond each specific treatment option, the most important message is that patients must recognize their own capacity to access opportunities if they choose to do so. Indeed, this realization is perhaps the greatest means of "stepping forward" to help oneself and one's family, and indeed to aid the scientific community in its reach toward curing this disease.

Christopher G. Goetz, MD
Professor of Neurological Sciences
Professor of Pharmacology
Rush University Medical Center
Chicago, Illinois

Introduction

This book was written using a previous book, *One Step at a Time*, as a foundation. The first two editions of *One Step at a Time* were written by my late father, who had twenty years of experience treating individuals with Parkinson's; my father and I co-wrote the third edition. This new book, *Parkinson's: Stepping Forward*, incorporates all of the treatment therapies and strategies for independence that *One Step at a Time* included. As well, I have added the latest research that contributes to our understanding of Parkinson's and its treatments. The language has been modified to make the book more user-friendly for patients and their caregivers, as well as those who treat Parkinson's.

The subtitle, *Stepping Forward*, is symbolic in many ways. Parkinson's research is advancing at a rapid pace and there are many new, positive developments. This is one forward step. Because of these advances, there are also many new strategies and treatments to improve the quality of life for people with Parkinson's. This is another forward step.

If you have Parkinson's, the most important thing is to keep a positive outlook. This will help you face your daily challenges, whether big or small, with greater ease. Your independence and your ability to exercise control over your activities are extremely valuable assets, not only to you but to those around you. This book will give you the information you need to keep Stepping Forward.

ONE

What Is Parkinson's?

At the age of sixty-two, Fred began to notice a constant aching pain in his right shoulder. Physiotherapy for a "frozen shoulder" provided some help, but the pain persisted. Six months later, his wife commented to him that she had started to notice that his right arm shook when he was sitting watching TV, and that he tended to walk without swinging that same arm.

Puzzled and a little worried, Fred reported his new symptoms to his doctor. After a thorough history and examination, his doctor offered a tentative diagnosis: "What I think we're seeing here, Fred, is the early stages of Parkinson's. I'm going to send you to a neurologist to see if he or she agrees; then we can decide on the best way to treat your symptoms. There are many different options available."

Parkinson's is a progressive disorder of the central nervous system. It is named after James Parkinson, a general practitioner in London, England, who was the first person to describe the clinical symptoms of "the shaking palsy," in a report published in 1817. In Parkinson's there is a loss of dopamine in the brain, which causes four main symptoms:

tremor, stiffness (rigidity), slow movements (bradykinesia), and loss of balance (postural instability).

Dopamine is a neurotransmitter, a chemical used by the brain to relay signals. When there is a loss of dopamine, the brain is not able to generate or transmit the proper signals to control movement. In the beginning, tremor and rigidity often occur on one side only.

Parkinson's is one of the most common neurological disorders, affecting 1 percent of adults over the age of sixty-five. The incidence is roughly the same in all countries around the world. It is more common in men, and usually begins between the ages of fifty and sixty-five, with an average age of onset of sixty. However, 5 to 10 percent of people with Parkinson's develop symptoms before the age of forty; this is called *young-onset* Parkinson's. Young-onset Parkinson's is basically the same illness as the older-onset type but with the following differences:

- The progression of parkinsonian signs and symptoms is more gradual.
- Motor complications from the medications tend to appear earlier.
- Memory disturbances and mental side effects of medications seem to develop later.
- Involuntary twisting or cramping of the foot (dystonia) is frequently present and is often among the first signs noticed.

Parkinson's can also develop under the age of twenty, in which case it is termed *juvenile onset*. Problems in a gene called parkin are now known to be the cause of the majority of these cases.

Once Parkinson's develops, the problem is usually slowly progressive—that is, it becomes worse. The rate of progress varies in different people, but most require treatment with a dopamine-replacing drug within two years of diagnosis. Some people, especially those with tremor of one arm, may have a very mild form and may require no treatment for a number of years. Overall, those who have tremor initially tend to have a milder type of Parkinson's.

The outlook for people with Parkinson's has improved markedly since the development of levodopa therapy in the early 1970s. (Levodopa is a dopamine-replacing drug.) Those who were previously confined to bed became mobile again. With modern drug therapy, disability is reduced at all stages and mortality is decreased. Unfortunately, no currently available therapies have been shown to have a major impact on the progression of the disease.

Types of Parkinsonism, and Disorders That May Be Confused with Parkinson's

The term "parkinsonism" refers to a group of disorders in which patients notice slow movements, stiffness of the limbs and difficulty walking. The most common slowly progressive condition that causes a parkinsonism is Parkinson's disease itself. However, essential tremor (tremor of unknown cause) is often misdiagnosed as Parkinson's disease, and a drug-induced form of parkinsonism is also very common. There is a large group of conditions that make up the other progressive parkinsonisms, which have been referred to in medical literature as atypical parkinsonism, pseudo-parkinsonism or Parkinson-plus. Parkinson's disease has also been called classic, idiopathic (meaning "cause not known"), primary or Lewy-body Parkinson's (a Lewy body is a round, microscopic structure found in brain cells at autopsy).

People with the classic signs and symptoms of rest tremor, unilateral (one-sided) stiffness and slowness of movements are normally very easily diagnosed. However, when people show other signs and symptoms it may take many months, or even years, before an accurate diagnosis can be made with certainty.

The most significant markers that someone may have Parkinson's are:

- symptoms beginning on one side
- rest tremor
- a clear, sustained response to dopamine-replacement therapy

Essential Tremor

Essential tremor is sometimes confused with Parkinson's, even though there are no symptoms other than tremor. Even the tremor itself is different. The tremor of Parkinson's occurs at rest, and stops or becomes less noticeable when movement is attempted. Essential tremor occurs when the hands are in a particular posture, such as holding a cup (postural tremor), or when the limb is moved toward an object (kinetic tremor). Other distinguishing features of essential tremor are:

- the presence of head tremor and sometimes voice tremor
- a family history of a similar tremor
- a longer history of tremor than in Parkinson's
- dramatic improvement of the tremor with small amounts of alcohol

People with essential tremor may also have some impairment of tandem walking (walking by placing one foot in front of the other). Essential tremor is much more common than Parkinson's and can occur at any age.

It is not always easy to distinguish essential tremor from Parkinson's; some people with Parkinson's also have a postural and kinetic tremor. In rare cases both conditions occur together. Some studies have raised the question of whether there is a link between essential tremor and Parkinson's, but there is no consensus on this at present. Treatments aimed at replacing dopamine loss are not effective for essential tremor, but it can be improved with either of two medications: propranolol or primidone.

Drug-Induced Parkinsonism

Many different kinds of medications have been reported to potentially cause a parkinson-like illness. The most common culprits in the past have been certain drugs used to treat serious mental illness. These drugs (*neuroleptics*) block dopamine receptors within the brain (see Chapter 2), so the brain doesn't have enough dopamine to adequately regulate the control or speed of movement.

Drug-induced parkinsonism is more likely to affect both sides of the body evenly, and is less likely to be associated with tremor. The condition usually develops in the first few months of drug use, but it can also start after the person has been on the drug for many years. Unlike the slow progression of true Parkinson's, significant disability may develop quite quickly in drug-induced parkinsonism, and the condition gets more severe the longer the drug is taken. Once the offending medication is stopped, most people recover within two months, but the problem can take over six months to resolve completely.

Drug-induced parkinsonism is seen more in older people, and it has been suggested that those who develop it may have a pre-existing brain dopamine deficiency. These patients have been shown to have various abnormalities in the dopamine-producing areas of the brain, which increase their risk of drug-induced parkinsonism.

There are many newer drugs for mental illnesses that are referred to as *atypical neuroleptics* because they are less likely to block the movement-related dopamine receptors in the brain. Although there is a smaller chance of these drugs causing drug-induced parkinsonism, it can still definitely happen—a fact which doctors sometimes overlook.

Some drugs used for stomach disorders can cause drug-induced parkinsonism. Metoclopramide is one; it is still frequently used in North America, and many physicians do not realize that it can cross into the brain and block dopamine. (Another similar medication called domperidone also blocks dopamine, but it cannot cross into the brain and therefore does not cause or worsen a parkinsonism.) Clebopride (available in Europe) has also been known to cause a parkinsonism.

Calcium-channel blockers, which are widely used for a number of illnesses (heart disease, high blood pressure) have the ability to interfere with dopamine transmission at many stages. Drugs of this class include diltiazem, nifedipine, verapamil, manipidine, captopril and amlodipine. These drugs could potentially worsen or cause a parkinsonism, but there is little evidence that they are directly involved. Considering the widespread use of these drugs for cardiovascular illness, and their benefits, anyone who has Parkinson's and is on a calcium-channel blocker must be carefully evaluated. (The situation is different with the calcium-channel blockers flunarizine and cinnarizine, which continue to be widely used in Mexico, Spain and South America; they have clearly been associated with a parkinsonism.)

Selective serotonin reuptake inhibitors (SSRIs) are drugs that increase another neurotransmitter, serotonin, in the brain. They are used to treat depression and anxiety. SSRIs include sertraline, paroxetine, fluvoxamine and fluoxetine.

A number of studies have suggested that SSRIs may cause a parkinsonism, or aggravate a pre-existing one. Most reports of such a parkinsonism involve the original drug in this class, fluoxetine. However, considering the small number of cases reported and the millions of people who have used this drug, the risk is extremely slight. It may be that other factors are involved—such as also being on another drug, selegiline. SSRIs are helpful and are normally well tolerated in depressed Parkinson's patients, but it should be remembered that there is a very low risk they could worsen the speed of function.

A number of other drugs have been reported to cause a parkinsonism in a few cases. These include meperidine (a pain medication), valproate (used to treat seizures), amiodarone (used for abnormal cardiac rhythms), vincristine and cytosine arabinoside (both anti-cancer drugs), lithium (a mood stabilizer), and alpha-methyldopa (an antidepressant).

The use of drugs that can block dopamine in the brain is also associated with a risk of developing unpleasant involuntary face and body movements (tardive dyskinesias). In anyone who has a parkinsonism, all drugs should be carefully reviewed, and the possibility of the parkinsonism being drug-induced should be considered and excluded.

Other Progressive Parkinsonisms
The illnesses that resemble Parkinson's are individually rare, but collectively these lookalikes may account for up to 20 percent of all cases of parkinsonism. Diagnosis of an atypical parkinsonism (a Parkinson-plus) is often difficult in the first few years of the illness, as the symptoms may result from any one of a number of disorders, and most of these disorders are of unknown cause.

However, it is important to try to identify the lookalike. An accurate diagnosis will allow a more definite prognosis (prediction of the future course of the disorder) and may avoid unnecessary drug costs and side effects. If someone has parkinsonian features with additional disabilities that are not seen regularly, or as severely, in classic Parkinson's, this may indicate that another illness is present.

These atypical disorders tend to cause earlier and more severe disability. The presence of some of the following fea-

tures may help differentiate them from Parkinson's:
- early onset and greater predominance of unsteady gait, postural defects and falls
- rapid progression
- absence of typical parkinsonian resting tremor
- early onset of memory problems
- atypical or severe stiffness with involuntary twisting movements
- early onset of dizziness associated with low blood pressure
- severe neck flexion (chin on chest)
- early onset of bladder dysfunction (often called neurogenic bladder) and sexual problems in both men and women
- abnormal reflexes on neurological exam
- impaired eye movements or eye opening
- poor or diminishing response to dopamine-replacement therapy

Because of the multiple problems that develop, people with these atypical disorders need careful assessment and follow-up care. Many things can be done to improve their comfort, mobility and quality of life.

The following are some of the conditions that may produce an atypical parkinsonism.

Progressive Supranuclear Palsy
This condition typically begins with gait problems and spontaneous backward falls, often in the first year of symptoms. It is more common in men. People with progressive supranuclear palsy are often unable to look down (although they may not be aware of this), and this causes problems walking, especially down stairs. Other eye problems may include:
- double vision
- blurred vision

- difficulty reading
- burning eyes
- light sensitivity
- slow eye opening and closing
- inability to open the eyes at will

Difficulty with speech and swallowing are common early in this disorder, as is the tendency for the eyes to close spontaneously (*blepharospasm*). There is not usually a significant rest tremor. Depression, slowed thinking, difficulty finding words, and reduced concentration occur in some people but not all. There is often a history of high blood pressure, and sleep upset with frequent wakenings. Progressive supranuclear palsy does slowly become worse, and unfortunately it does not respond to drugs as well as typical Parkinson's does. However, blepharospasm may respond well to local injections of botulinum toxin into the eyelid muscles.

Multiple System Atrophy
Of the atypical parkinsonisms, multiple system atrophy can be the hardest to distinguish from Parkinson's. The initial symptoms are:
- slowness
- unsteadiness
- walking difficulty
- bladder and sexual problems
- lightheadedness on standing up

Only about 5 percent of people with multiple system atrophy have early tremor. Rest tremor is rarely present, although many individuals have other types of tremor. Additional problems that may develop are:
- low-volume voice

- excess saliva
- swallowing difficulty
- poor handwriting
- bowel dysfunction
- respiratory dysfunction

Blood pressure often becomes a major problem, as the drop in blood pressure that occurs upon standing up may cause unconsciousness. Dopamine-replacement medications make this drop in blood pressure worse. Often the blood pressure increases when the person lies down, so he or she appears to have hypertension (high blood pressure) and may be put on antihypertensive medication, which further lowers the standing blood pressure. For this reason, anyone suspected of having multiple system atrophy should always have blood pressure checked both lying down and standing up.

Multiple system atrophy often shows some response to levodopa, but the person is frequently more disabled by poor balance than by slowness. Some people have no motor response to levodopa, yet develop excessive involuntary movements (dyskinesias).

In the past, multiple system atrophy was separated into three supposedly distinct conditions, but it was increasingly recognized that the categories frequently overlapped. If the person had more stiffness and no tremor, the term *striatonigral degeneration* was used. If prominent early unsteadiness was one of the main features, the term *olivopontocerebellar degeneration* was used. If, in addition, there were prominent early sexual dysfunction and blood pressure drops on standing, the term *Shy-Drager syndrome* was used.

Corticobasal Degeneration (CBD)
This is an uncommon disorder that causes marked stiffness,

complex sensory defects (such as not being able to recognize an object placed in one's hand) and jerky movements, starting on only one side of the body, in classic cases. Many people with CBD also have significant memory difficulties. Treatment is difficult, as there is little response to dopamine-replacement therapies, but the jerky movements can be modestly improved with clonazepam.

Parkinsonism and Prominent Memory Difficulties

In a number of different conditions, a parkinsonism is associated with prominent memory and thinking difficulties (*dementia*).

Alzheimer's Disease

One-third of people with Alzheimer's also have rigidity and slowness that suggest Parkinson's, although they have little tremor and their symptoms do not respond well to dopamine-replacement therapies. The slowness of movement normally develops many years after the onset of the memory difficulties.

Dementia with Lewy Bodies

Dementia with Lewy bodies (also called diffuse Lewy-body disease) was once thought to be rare but is now felt to account for at least 25 percent of elderly demented individuals. The main signs and symptoms are:
- visual hallucinations
- fluctuating confusion
- agitation
- parkinsonism

In autopsies of people with Parkinson's disease, Lewy bodies are seen in the substantia nigra (a structure found at the top of the spinal cord). They are one of the key features that confirm the diagnosis. Some people have these structures all through the brain (cerebral cortex), hence the name *diffuse* Lewy-body disease, or dementia with Lewy bodies. In these people the features of parkinsonism are seen early, and are more prominent than in people with Alzheimer's. Individuals with diffuse Lewy bodies frequently have depression, increased daytime sleepiness and night upsets, including muscle jerks and violent behavior. Hallucinations and varying behavior over the course of the day are the hallmark of this problem. Although the current guidelines for diagnosing this condition state that the memory difficulties should start within one year of the parkinsonism, there are many reports of people who followed the typical course of Parkinson's disease, without significant memory difficulties, for more than ten years, yet were found at autopsy to have Lewy bodies throughout the brain. This has created controversy as to the relationship between the two conditions, and whether they are truly separate disorders.

Frontotemporal dementia
This dementia, affecting the frontal and temporal lobes of the brain, is less common but it too may be confused with Parkinson's. The cause of this form of dementia is unknown. It causes profound personality change, poor social conduct, and lack of motivation and insight. However, some people retain fairly intact memory. Others have progressive speech difficulty, with problems understanding, but their memory function is relatively well preserved. In this condition any parkinsonism is normally mild, and occurs very late if it occurs at all.

Vascular Parkinsonism
This condition typically involves the legs more than the arms. An early sign is a stiff, slow, short-stepped walk (lower-body parkinsonism) that may begin fairly suddenly. Vascular parkin-

sonism is caused by multiple small strokes, and is seen in people with high blood pressure, heart disease and/or poor circulation in their feet. Usually there is no tremor, and the response to dopamine-replacement therapies is poor. An imaging test of the brain (CT or MRI scan) is very useful in confirming this diagnosis. Care must be taken not to overinterpret these brain scans, though, as many people over the age of sixty show small changes, without having a vascular parkinsonism.

Post-Traumatic Parkinsonism

This is seen in boxers, and is related to the number of bouts fought, not to the number of knockouts. In addition to variable signs of parkinsonism, people with post-traumatic parkinsonism have memory and behavioral upsets. The disorder may begin decades after the last fight, and is rarely seen after a single severe head injury. It is thought that the repeated blows to the head suffered in boxing cause damage to the substantia nigra. Some studies have suggested that minor head trauma may be a risk factor for the development of Parkinson's, but this remains controversial. The condition responds to medication less predictably than does typical Parkinson's.

Wilson's Disease

Anyone under the age of fifty who shows symptoms of parkinsonism (stiffness, slowness, tremor) should be tested for this rare genetic defect, as the condition is treatable. Because of a defect in copper metabolism, copper deposits appear in the liver, brain and corneas of the eyes. The disease normally starts during childhood or adolescence, and has only rarely been reported as starting in someone over the age of fifty.

No one test is 100 percent sensitive or specific for Wilson's disease, so multiple screening tests are required, taking a close look at the cornea, and checking blood and a twenty-four-hour urine collection. In someone who has the disorder, blood and urine tests will show increased copper, and a low blood level of a copper transport protein (*ceruloplasmin*). An MRI scan of the brain will often show density changes in the basal ganglia. The gene defect for Wilson's disease has been identified, and DNA testing can help confirm the diagnosis if the basic tests are positive. At the present time this testing is difficult to perform and is done only in research laboratories, so most people will not have the procedure. A liver biopsy is sometimes necessary, when the results of screening tests are inconclusive or conflicting.

Parkinsonism with Hydrocephalus (Normal Pressure Hydrocephalus)

Within the middle of the brain are fluid-filled structures called *ventricles*. In this form of parkinsonism, the ventricles enlarge (called *hydrocephalus*). This condition is rare, and is diagnosed with the help of a CT or MRI brain scan. The person has prominent memory loss, usually without tremor, difficulties with unsteady walking and poor bladder control. The treatment of this condition is complex, and unfortunately the surgery to reduce the abnormally large cavities is not always successful.

TWO

The cause of Parkinson's is not fully understood. However, we have known for more than thirty years that the main symptoms of Parkinson's are due to a deficiency in the production of the neurotransmitter dopamine. Why does a loss of dopamine cause such a range of physical problems?

Consider how the brain controls physical movement.

Dopamine and the Healthy Brain

The main body of the brain has various lobes that control many of our perceptions and abilities, including memory, spatial judgment, language and so on. Buried within the right and left sides of this main part of the brain is a region called the basal ganglia. One of the main functions of the basal ganglia is to enable us to perform smooth, dexterous movements.

The basal ganglia are made up of complex groups of cells subdivided into the *caudate, putamen, globus pallidus, subthalamic nucleus* and *substantia nigra*. The substantia nigra is the deepest structure, located around the top of the spine in a more primitive area called the *brainstem*. (Like most parts of the brain, all of these groups of cells are found on both the

Anatomy of the brain

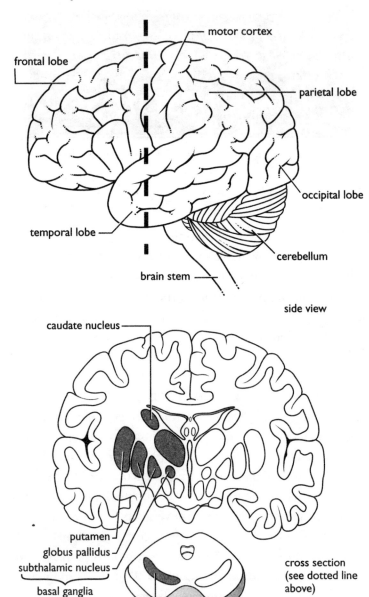

frontal lobe

motor cortex

parietal lobe

occipital lobe

temporal lobe

cerebellum

brain stem

side view

caudate nucleus

putamen
globus pallidus
subthalamic nucleus
basal ganglia

substantia nigra

brain stem

cross section
(see dotted line
above)

right and left sides of the brain.) The names of these structures can get very confusing, as different combinations of structures have additional names; for example, the caudate and putamen are often referred to jointly as the *striatum*. The caudate and putamen receive input from the outside lobes of the brain, as well as from the substantia nigra.

Dopamine is produced within the substantia nigra, and is the neurotransmitter (chemical messenger) used to send signals from the substantia nigra up to the caudate and putamen.

How Brain Cells Communicate

The main cells within the brain that are involved in sending signals to other parts of the brain are called *neurons*. Each neuron has a cell wall and a nucleus, just like many other cells in the body. Each neuron also has a main tube called an *axon*, that extends out to send information to other cells within the brain and spinal cord. Often the end of axon doesn't just connect to one cell, but divides into many small finger-like extensions to connect to hundreds and sometimes thousands of other neurons.

There is no direct connection between the cells; instead there is a very small gap between them called a *synapse*. One cell therefore has to send its information across this small gap to reach the other cell. Neurotransmitters are the chemical messengers used to carry the information across the synapse. The brain uses many different neurotransmitters to send signals from cell to cell, including dopamine, acetylcholine, serotonin and norepinephrine.

What Goes Wrong in Parkinson's?

When the dopamine-producing cells in the substantia nigra die, the caudate and putamen areas of the basal ganglia become deficient in dopamine. This causes the other parts of the basal ganglia to become unregulated, resulting in the various problems of physical control that we call Parkinson's. These problems begin to be seen when at least 60 percent of the dopamine-producing neurons of the substantia nigra have been lost, and there is more than a 60 percent reduction in dopamine in the basal ganglia.

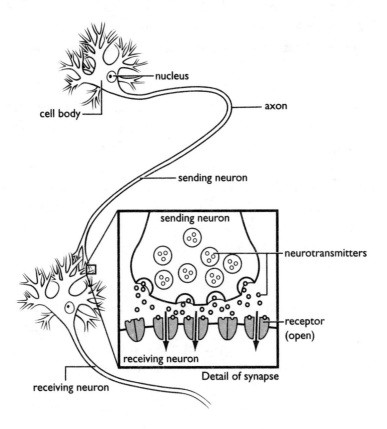

Neurons and a synapse

Why Do Dopamine-Producing Cells Die?

Unfortunately, we are still not sure why this happens. Many potential factors are being actively investigated, including:

- deficiencies in a cell's ability to clear toxins
- energy failure within the neurons
- a "programmed suicide" mechanism called *apoptosis*
- deficiencies of growth factors
- a neuron's inability to properly clear proteins
- an accelerated aging process
- inflammation
- factors related to the immune process, which normally protects the body against infection

Toxic exposure for cells can come not only from substances from outside the body, but also from ones produced within the body. All the cells in the body have to make their own energy, to survive and function properly. They use oxygen to produce energy, and toxic substances are byproducts of this process. The toxic byproducts created by this energy-producing process have to be cleared very efficiently, or they may kill the cell. The whole process places the cell under "oxidative" stress.

Researchers into Parkinson's have studied this toxic mechanism in detail for more than twenty years. There is clear evidence that the process is not functioning normally in people with Parkinson's, but it's not clear if this is the primary cause of cell death or just a secondary reaction to another problem.

If a cell could not produce its own energy this would also lead to the cell's death. In Parkinson's, there is evidence that the energy-producing part of the cell is not working properly—but, again, this could be secondary to another process going wrong first.

All cells are capable of undergoing a programmed suicide, or apoptosis, and how this process works within the cell has become better understood in the last few years. During the development of the brain of a fetus, many extra cells are produced, which must then die once the proper connections are formed.

The cells achieve this by turning on their apoptosis genes. There is evidence that in Parkinson's the dopamine-producing cells in the brain are dying by this process. The genes and chemicals involved in controlling apoptosis are now being identified.

The identification of specific gene abnormalities in rare individuals with Parkinson's has suggested another potential mechanism for cell death. Proteins are continuously being made in cells, and once they have completed their job they must be disposed of. If a cell cannot clear the protein properly, the protein will start to accumulate in the cell, with potentially harmful consequences. These abnormal protein-clearance pathways are just beginning to be understood. In the future we may be able to develop drugs that block these pathways.

Many neurological diseases appear to be related to problems of the immune system. An infection by a virus which then activates the immune system has been suggested as a possible trigger for the neurological disease. However, in Parkinson's there is very little evidence that this occurs. Another possibility that researchers are beginning to explore is that some growth factor the brain cells normally produce to survive may be lacking. This theory still requires a lot more background work, but the potential of using growth factors as a treatment for Parkinson's is already being examined. What might trigger any of these processes is unclear, but both environmental and genetic factors have been implicated.

Parkinson's and Genetics
This has been one of the most exciting and active areas of Parkinson's research in the last few years. The recent identification of single-gene defects in people with some form of Parkinson's gives tremendous hope for understanding its cause. Genes contain the information that decide an individual's characteristics, including things like eye and hair color. Genes also

control the production of proteins, and these proteins have many functions in normal cells. Some are vital elements in the production of brain chemicals such as dopamine. If a gene is abnormal, the proteins produced are also not normal, and vital cell functions may slow down, leading eventually to cell death.

With modern tools of molecular biology and molecular genetics, there have been many exciting advances in this field. It takes time, however, to identify specific genes and their abnormalities. Once the gene has been identified, its function must be understood, and then therapies must be developed and tested to either change or compensate for the abnormal function. Although each step, from gene identification to understanding and altering functions, takes years of work, we can hope that new approaches to prevention and treatment will open up in the not too distant future. These strategies may include adding a gene that increases or decreases the production of specific proteins to help save the dopamine cells.

There is increasing evidence that genetic factors play a role in causing Parkinson's. Apart from age, a positive family history of Parkinson's is the strongest predictor of an increased risk of developing the disease. A common way to try to determine whether there is a genetic component to a disease is to study twins. Identical twins share the same genes but nonidentical twins share only half their genes. If a disease has a strong genetic component, there will be more sets of identical twins than non-identical twins in which both twins are affected by the disease. Studies of sets of twins support the concept of a genetic component in Parkinson's, especially among people whose disease appears before the age of fifty.

When someone in a family is affected by Parkinson's, the increased risk of another family member developing it is small. However, in a few families with multiple affected individuals there is up to a 50 percent chance of the other close relatives developing Parkinson's. In some of these families, a specific genetic change (mutation) has been identified that causes their disease. A defect in a gene called alpha-synuclein was originally found in a large Italian family and three Greek families. A different defect within the same gene was found in one German family. To date, only eight families have been found to have alpha-synuclein gene defects and Parkinson's, despite thousands of patients being screened for the combination, suggesting that such defects are an extremely rare cause of Parkinson's. However, this discovery has given us important insights into the basic mechanisms of the disease. Lewy bodies (those microscopic round structures found in brain cells affected by Parkinson's) have been found to have a high concentration of alpha-synuclein. Animal models of Parkinson's that have had gene manipulations to change the function of alpha-synuclein are now being studied. These new animal models have changed our ideas about how Parkinson's may develop. It is now suspected that the mutation in alpha-synuclein leads to an accumulation of protein, which forms the Lewy body as well as disrupting the function of the dopamine-producing neurons.

The list of genes that have been identified as causing Parkinson's is rapidly expanding, and currently includes not only alpha-synuclein but also parkin, ubiquitin carboxy terminal hydrolase-L1, DJ1 and the NR4A2 genes. Over the next few years more such genes will almost surely be found. Mutations in the parkin gene were originally described in Japanese patients with a very early onset of symptoms, and parkin mutations are now recognized as causing Parkinson's in the majority of individuals whose disease begins before the age of twenty. (This juvenile Parkinson's is very uncommon.) Mutations in parkin have been identified in people over the age of sixty, but in very few cases. Mutations in ubiquitin carboxy terminal hydrolase-L1 genes have been found in only one family to date. The DJ1 and NR4A2 genes have just been reported, and wider screening for mutations in these genes is underway, but we do not yet know how common they may be.

Although we still don't know how these newly identified genes in these rare families relate to most people with Parkinson's, they will at the very least provide important clues to further our understanding of the mechanisms involved. According to our present knowledge about most families, the pattern of inheritance is not strong enough or clear enough that people with Parkinson's should be unduly worried about their children developing the disease. At present there is no simple test for Parkinson's; genetic testing is being done only in research laboratories, and is not commercially available.

Environmental Toxin Exposure

As we age, we all slowly lose our dopamine-producing cells. Perhaps the development of Parkinson's is the result of an event earlier in life that killed a portion of these cells. With some cells already gone, symptoms would show up many years later, when cell loss reached a critical level because of the further loss that is part of the normal aging process.

This hypothetical event killing off cells earlier in life might be exposure to some environmental toxin. It is now known that certain specific toxins such as MPTP can precipitate Parkinson's. (MPTP was made by accident by some IV drug users trying to create hallucinogenic street drugs.) These types of toxins are rare, and it is very unlikely that most people will have any exposure to them.

Parkinson's has been shown in some studies to be more common in farming and/or rural communities, in people who drink well water and in those who have had a higher exposure to pesticides. All this suggests that some environmental toxic agents could be causing the increased risk. There have been many attempts to identify more common toxins that could increase this risk, but to date no specific ones have been

---

The question of iron

We know that there is excess iron in the brains of people with Parkinson's. As well, there are some abnormalities in the ways their bodies and brains handle iron. Although it has been suggested that iron may be an important issue in the disorder, the prevailing opinion is that it is not a primary factor in causing Parkinson's.

---

found. Interestingly, smoking seems to give some protection against the development of Parkinson's. It is unclear why this could be so, and in view of the many harmful effects of smoking, no one would recommend starting to smoke to decrease the chance of developing Parkinson's.

How Is Parkinson's Diagnosed?

Special diagnostic tests are rarely helpful in confirming the diagnosis of either typical Parkinson's or one of the atypical forms of parkinsonism. Instead, a diagnosis of Parkinson's is usually made on the basis of clinical observations by an experienced neurologist.

If there are unusual symptoms, or if the response to medication is poor, the following special diagnostic tests may be used to scan the brain:

- computerized tomography (CT) scan
- magnetic resonance imaging (MRI) scan
- positron emission tomography (PET) scan
- single photon emission computed tomography (SPECT) scan
- ultrasound

Computerized Tomography (CT) Scans

A CT scan will show normal results in someone with typical Parkinson's. However, a CT scan can show other brain conditions, such as hydrocephalus (the enlargement of fluid-filled cavities in the brain) and tissue damage from small strokes (which interrupt the blood flow to some part of the brain, causing brain tissue to die from lack of oxygen). A CT scan takes X-ray pictures of the brain and assembles them into a two-dimensional image. The process is not painful or invasive, but it involves lying with the head inside a hollow tube; some people find this claustrophobic.

Magnetic Resonance Imaging (MRI) Scans

MRI scanning can be helpful in diagnosing atypical and pseudo-parkinsonism conditions, and in patients with unsatisfactory response to drugs. In multiple system atrophy, an MRI scan may show smallness of the brainstem (also seen in progressive supranuclear palsy); smallness of the cerebellum (which controls balance); and changes in the putamen. MRI scans can also show hydrocephalus, small strokes and the basal ganglia changes of Wilson's disease.

MRI scans do not use X-rays. Instead, they track the minute energy changes that appear when brain tissue is briefly exposed to a powerful magnetic field. Like a CT scan, an MRI scan is not painful but may be claustrophobic. MRI scans cannot be done on people who have any metal fragments in their heads or eyes, from welding, for example.

A new kind of MRI scanning that is becoming more widely available is called MRI spectroscopy. Spectroscopy is a refinement of MRI and can show some aspects of cell function. Investigators are finding some promising indications that this type of scanning may be useful to help differentiate atypical parkinsonisms from Parkinson's. This technique is still considered a research tool; further studies will show whether it is truly useful.

PET and SPECT Scans

Positive emission tomography (PET) and single photon emission computed tomography (SPECT) scans are also still research tools that are being refined. In these tests, radioactive markers are injected into the person and then, a few hours to one day later, a scan is done. This test is also not uncomfortable, aside from the injection, and simply requires lying down. The radioactive exposure is extremely small. To test for Parkinson's, the radioactive markers are designed to attach themselves to the dopamine cells in the brain, and the SPECT or PET scanner then measures the amount of attachment. Because both Parkinson's and atypical parkinsonism are associated with a loss of dopamine, the attachment is measurably less.

These new brain-imaging techniques are likely to become important in providing a more definite early diagnosis, and in allowing us to monitor the results of treatment. They will also be crucial in testing *neuroprotective* therapies, which are meant to slow or stop the progression of Parkinson's.

PET scanning is very expensive and not widely available. However, most hospitals have equipment that can perform SPECT scans.

Ultrasound

Ultrasound scanning has been used for a long time to assess areas of the body that are not covered by bone. For example, this type of scanning is frequently used to look for abnormalities in the abdomen (kidneys, gallbladder or intestines), and is used to assess the fetus during pregnancy. A probe is held over the area of interest and specific sound waves are directed through the skin. When the sound waves "hit" different structures the sound is reflected and recorded by the probe. Ultrasound has not been used in the past for problems with the brain because the hard bony skull would block the sound waves. New refinements in this technology are now allowing us to image the substantia nigra area. Differences in how the sound waves are reflected have been reported in individuals with Parkinson's, compared to people without symptoms or with some of the atypical parkinsonisms. Ultrasound scanning machines are widely available and inexpensive to run, and in the future this may be an easy way to help confirm the diagnosis of Parkinson's.

THREE

How Does Parkinson's Affect You?

People with Parkinson's may experience a wide range of symptoms, both major and minor. Some of these problems are caused by the disorder itself. Others are side effects of various medications. For practical tips on dealing with these issues, see Chapter 4. But remember—while the list of possible problems may look daunting, nobody has all of these.

Medications used for Parkinson's are discussed in detail in Chapter 6, and are listed in a table at the back of the book. However, it's helpful to have some familiarity with the main types of medication, to understand some of their benefits and side effects.

Levodopa (L-dopa) is converted to dopamine in the brain. Since people with Parkinson's are deficient in dopamine, most people with the disorder will eventually take levodopa. However, while it's the best treatment we have at present, it does have a number of troublesome side effects.

Amantadine can be helpful in the early as well as late stages of Parkinson's, but we don't know exactly how it works.

Dopamine agonists mimic the effects of dopamine by stimulating the dopamine receptors in the brain. They too have possible side effects, and are used in early or late stages of the disease.

Monoamine oxidase inhibitors (MAOIs) include selegiline, a drug that inactivates the breakdown of dopamine within the brain. Selegiline has typically been used mostly in the early stages of the disease.

Anticholinergics block a brain neurotransmitter called acetylcholine. This is thought to restore a more normal balance between acetylcholine and dopamine. Anticholinergics can be used to reduce tremor, but they tend to cause confusion and memory problems, especially in older people.

Main Symptoms

Four symptoms and signs—tremor, rigidity, bradykinesia and postural instability—are the main clinical features used to make a diagnosis of Parkinson's. Not every person has all of the features, especially at the beginning of the course of the disease. The earliest complaints may include fatigue, a general feeling of weakness, small handwriting, poor hand coordination and a tremulous feeling in one arm, with or without observable tremor.

Tremor

Since retiring, George had enjoyed watching TV in the afternoons. In the last couple of months, though, he had noticed that his right thumb was twitching on its own while he sat quietly in his chair. Now he found that his whole right hand was beginning to shake.

Tremor is a rhythmic involuntary movement that normally affects the hand but can also involve the foot or jaw. Tremor is caused by the alternating contraction of opposed muscle groups, so that the affected body part is jerked first one way and then the other. This can be the most bothersome of all the symptoms, but it is normally the least disabling. The most common tremor is a movement of the thumb and first finger, giving a pill-rolling effect.

People with Parkinson's typically have a resting tremor—that is, the tremor ceases when they reach out or perform some activity. A postural tremor (e.g., when holding your hands extended in front of you) and/or a kinetic tremor (beginning when you move) can accompany resting tremor, but is not typical of the disorder (see "Essential Tremor," Chapter 1).

Resting tremor is seen at some stage in most cases of Parkinson's, but it is important to remember that up to one-third of people with Parkinson's do not have this symptom. It is infrequent in the disorders that mimic Parkinson's. People whose Parkinson's begins with tremor tend to have a milder course of the illness. Some people with Parkinson's have a feeling of tremor inside their chest, abdomen or limbs, but no tremor is seen by an observer.

Rigidity

Rigidity refers to muscular stiffness, and increased muscle resistance to passive movement of joints when the limb is relaxed. (Passive movement is movement applied by another person—for example, by a doctor or therapist gently bending the wrist, turning the head or flexing the elbow.) The person with Parkinson's is usually not aware of the rigidity, but is troubled by muscle slowness. Rigidity is not as specific to Parkinson's as a resting tremor, and is more apparent to the examining doctor than to the patient.

Bradykinesia

People with bradykinesia—slowness of movement—take longer to complete an activity. This means that it may take them more time and effort to perform the normal routines of daily living. As well, the movements associated with an activity are reduced. For example, they may swing their arms less when walking, or not cross their legs when sitting. They may also have slower facial movements, or reduced eye blinking, which can result in a mask-like or staring expression.

Bradykinesia tends to cause more disability than either tremor or rigidity, but fortunately this is the symptom that responds best to currently available treatments. The degree of bradykinesia is tested by observing the slowness of the person rising from a chair, and the slowness and difficulty he or she has in sustaining quick alternating movements (e.g., rapid finger-to-thumb closing, or rapid opening and closing of a fist). Difficulty turning in bed is another symptom that is caused by bradykinesia.

Postural Instability
We normally keep our balance without really thinking about it, because our reflexes make small adjustments to our position to keep us upright. The progressive decline of these postural reflexes, leading to a loss of balance, is probably the most disabling of all parkinsonian symptoms.

Walking and turning are unsteady, and sometimes the person falls. The degree of instability is tested by observing the person's response to a sudden pull on the shoulders from behind. Someone without Parkinson's will take a step backwards, while someone with more advanced Parkinson's, with postural instability, will be unable to recover and will fall backwards.

The instability becomes more prevalent as the illness progresses; if it is present early, this suggests that the problem may be something other than Parkinson's.

Scales for Rating Disability

There are many different scales for determining the degree of disability in a person with Parkinson's. They include the Unified Parkinson Disease Rating Scale (UPDRS), the Hoehn and Yahr Scale, and the Schwab and England Scale. These scales are used by clinic nurses and neurologists to assess and document changes in the person's condition over the long term. In the short term, however, people may find that their level of mobility fluctuates drastically from day to day, or even during the course of the day—particularly once their Parkinson's is advanced.

Unified Parkinson Disease Rating Scale

UPDRS is a very detailed and extensive scoring system that evaluates more than forty different aspects of Parkinson's, including depression, swallowing, dressing and gait. It is the scale most commonly used to assess people with Parkinson's in clinical research trials.

Hoehn and Yahr Scale

According to this scale, there are five stages of parkinsonian disability, judged by the major symptoms listed above. The scale reflects increasing disease severity, but it is not a good indicator of the more continuous progression of the disease. For example, many people spend most of the time in stages I to III and less time in stages IV and V.

Stage I
One-sided tremor or rigidity with or without slowness of movement. Mildly affected patients at stage I may not need any treatment, but those with moderate disability will be much more comfortable with therapy.

Stage II
Moderate tremor or rigidity on both sides, with bradykinesia.

Symptoms will be improved by the use of levodopa or amantadine, or dopamine agonists.

Stage III
Significant tremor, rigidity and/or bradykinesia, accompanied by mobility problems. Difficulties in postural control develop; there is unsteadiness on turns, and hesitations, halts and freezes when starting to walk. Patients may begin to notice fluctuations in their level of function within the day, and may experience dyskinesias (drug-induced involuntary movements). The major new problem at this stage is balance difficulty.

Stage IV
More severe disability, but still able to walk. Bradykinesia is more severe and patients require some assistance with activities of daily living. If there are fluctuations in the level of function, they too will be more severe.

Stage V
Loss of ability to function independently. Postural defects are severe and independent mobility is impossible.

Schwab and England Scale
The Schwab and England Scale is used to assess someone's level of independence.

100% Completely independent. Able to do all chores without slowness, difficulty or impairment. Essentially normal. Unaware of any difficulty.

90% Completely independent. Able to do all chores with some degree of slowness, difficulty and impairment; may take twice as long. Beginning to be aware of difficulty.

80% Completely independent in most chores. Takes twice as long. Conscious of difficulty and slowness.

On and off

A person's response to dopamine-replacement drugs may vary from one time to another. We say the person is in an "on" period when the drugs are working and movements are easier, and in an "off" period when the drugs are not working and movements are more difficult.

70% Not completely independent. More difficulty with some chores. Three to four times as long in doing some. Must spend a large part of the day on chores.

60% Some dependency. Can do most chores, but exceedingly slowly and with much effort. Errors are made; some tasks are impossible.

50% More dependent. Needs help with half the chores, showering, bathing, etc. Difficulty with everything.

40% Very dependent. Can assist with all chores, but can do few alone.

30% With effort, now and then does a few chores alone, or begins alone. Much help needed.

20% Nothing alone. Can be a slight help with some chores. Severe invalid.

10% Totally dependent, helpless. Complete invalid.

People whose mobility fluctuates severely may vary greatly from one time to another. For example, someone who functions at 75 percent during a good or "on" period may revert to a 25 percent level during a bad or "off" period. Note, too, that not everyone experiences the more severe stages.

Other Problems

In addition to the major impairments listed above, a host of other signs and symptoms may develop in the course of the disorder. Some of them are common; some are fairly rare.

Gait Difficulties

Walking problems are common in Parkinson's and can be a source of great frustration. The problems may be related to slowness of movement (bradykinesia), and may respond well to medication; or they may be secondary to loss of balance (postural instability), which results from other changes in the basal ganglia, brainstem and/or frontal lobes, in which case they will not improve with drug treatment. The following may also contribute to walking problems:

- foot cramping
- hip and knee arthritis
- severe spinal-disc disease
- memory and thinking problems

Whatever the causes, walking problems can lead to a cautious gait and a loss of confidence. When the problems are mild, people can adapt to them. As disability increases, they may have great problems starting to walk (*start hesitation*), especially from low chairs; they may also get their feet tangled on turns, and lose their balance. In addition, they notice that walking now requires much more conscious effort—and this effort is in turn more difficult if their thinking is slowed.

In a normal walking pattern, the heel strikes the floor first. After this disability has been present for some time, the pattern is reversed and a toe-first walk develops. The length of stride is reduced and a shuffling gait develops. Turning is slower, and the feet drag, causing noise. Some people have brief halts and stalls called *freezing*. Arm swing may be decreased and hand tremor may increase during walking.

Cognitive Impairment

Disorders of cognition—of thinking and understanding—

affect a large percentage of people with Parkinson's. They can be even more disabling than the motor (movement) difficulties. They may be part of the illness, or may result from treatment.

Serious cognitive impairment, known as dementia, involves the loss of such mental functions as memory, judgment and reasoning. It is estimated that about 45 percent of those with Parkinson's will have some impairment of their cognitive function. Of these, about half will be more severely affected, by dementia. Dementia and delirium—severe, often frenzied confusion—are the leading reasons for people with Parkinson's being placed in nursing homes.

Mild impairment may not be recognized; people just appear more passive and seem to have less energy. They deny that they are depressed, they don't have guilt feelings (a common symptom of depression) and they don't usually respond to antidepressant medications. They have some slowing of memory and information processing but they may not fully appreciate their problem. These people are at more risk of developing delirium if they are treated with dopamine-replacement medications than are people with Parkinson's who do not have memory difficulties.

Memory Disorders and Dementia

Janice was in her seventies and had had Parkinson's for the last ten years. She noticed that she was having more trouble remembering her grocery list these days, and was tending to misplace her car keys. It seemed to her that she was having more memory problems than her friends of the same age. However, she found that by writing more lists, and generally working harder at being organized, she could continue to function independently.

Anticholinergics and amantadine, used to treat early Parkinson's, can cause cognitive difficulty. Some of the new drugs used to treat memory loss are starting to be used for this mild impairment as well. For the majority of people with Parkinson's, however, mild memory loss has little impact on the activities of daily living. Remember that mild impairment is common as people age, even when they don't have a neurological disease.

The more severe impairment of dementia is a major problem, and it significantly changes the way the Parkinson's is managed, as drug treatment may easily lead to delirium. The severe memory loss of Parkinson-related dementia is seen more in older people, those with greater motor impairment, and those with a family history of memory problems.

Dementia is uncommon in the first five years of the illness; indeed, if it is present early, the disorder may not be typical Parkinson's.

Depression may at times be confused with memory loss, regardless of whether the person has Parkinson's or not. It's important that the depression be recognized, as depression is readily treatable.

Confusion and Hallucinations

Andy had had Parkinson's for a long time. In the last few years he had clearly been having more difficulty with his memory. He was starting to notice a tendency to "see" things that he knew shouldn't be there, especially at night. He would look at the curtains and think he saw a person in the room. When he got up to go to the washroom, he would think he saw bugs on the floor.

At first Andy was quite frightened, but then he realized that these were simply illusions and hallucinations. He discussed the problem with his doctor, who changed his dopamine-replacement medication, and the phantom images went away.

In up to one-third of people with late-stage Parkinson's—most commonly those whose memories are impaired—drug treatment leads to confusion and hallucinations. (If the confusion and hallucinations begin before drugs are started, the person may not have typical Parkinson's; confusion and hallucinations are often the first symptom of diffuse Lewy-body disease.)

Any of the drugs used to treat Parkinson's may cause confusion or perceptual changes. People may have difficulty with memory or reasoning. Perceptual changes may consist of illusions, in which objects are mistaken for something else, and hallucinations, in which non-existent people, animals or objects are seen. If the problem is severe, there may be manic (uncontrollable) behavior, hypersexuality (exaggerated sexual behavior) and paranoid psychosis. (The term "psychosis" is used if the hallucinations and delusions are persistent.)

Although hallucinations can affect any of the senses—vision, smell, touch, taste or hearing—visual hallucinations are the most common. Some people experience the sensation of seeing ill-defined things at the side of their vision. This is also a drug effect, but it's not as serious or upsetting as hallucinations. Some older people with impaired vision have quite benign visual hallucinations.

More often, though, hallucinations are a serious and unpleasant problem; indeed, they are a common reason for people being placed in a nursing home. Someone who develops hallucinations may need medication that specifically treats the hallucinations, or may need a reduction of the medication already being given.

Vivid dreaming or nightmares may be an early sign of side effects caused by medications; later, the dreams may become more severe and frequent. Levodopa, amantadine, dopamine agonists, anticholinergics or the MAOI drug selegiline may all cause these effects.

Almost any drug may worsen the confusion of a person with a parkinsonism: pain medication, minor tranquilizers, antidepressants, even drugs to reduce stomach acid. If the problem comes on suddenly, the doctor may reduce the drug doses significantly for a few days or a week, and then use a lower dosage, or change to another drug altogether. In people with advanced Parkinson's, the hallucinations or confusion are more difficult to control and may actually limit the drug treatment. People may prefer to accept mild confusion and illusions if it allows them better mobility.

Emotional Problems

Depression
Common indications that someone with Parkinson's may be experiencing depression include:
- worsened sleep, with early-morning wakening
- complaints of a decrease in memory
- a decrease in appetite, although older patients may eat more
- more slowness of movement, tremor or walking difficulties
- loss of energy and interest; sadness, crying
- feelings of guilt and helplessness

Maureen had been struggling with her recent diagnosis of Parkinson's. Her doctor insisted that her new medication would help her function better, and was convinced that her walking and other movements had improved since her previous appointment. But Maureen said she felt worse than ever.

With further discussion, they both realized that Maureen's lack of response was due to depression. Once the depression was treated, she regained her active, enjoyable lifestyle.

People are more likely to suffer significant depression if they have impaired memory and are substantially disabled, but depression may also appear before the physical symptoms of parkinsonism. It may be a major factor in someone's perceived lack of response to dopamine-replacement therapy. Sometimes, the depression is recognized when the physician can see that the patient has clear functional improvement, but the patient denies that anything has improved.

Anxiety and Panic Attacks
Although most of us experience anxiety at some time in our lives, about 40 percent of people with Parkinson's experience anxiety, with or without panic attacks, that significantly affects their functioning. When panic attacks appear, they are associated with dizziness, shortness of breath and sweating.

Agitation
Agitation may be brought on by antiparkinson drugs, or it may be a reaction to the Parkinson's itself. It can manifest itself as fidgeting, poor concentration or changes in behavior. It is more common in those whose memories are impaired.

Fatigue
Fatigue is a common symptom in Parkinson's, and it may be a very prominent and disabling complaint. It is not always associated with more severe disability, sleep disturbance or medication effect; it is also seen in people who are only mildly disabled. There is currently much discussion as to whether the fatigue originates from the shortage of dopamine in the brain or from the loss of other neurotransmitters in the brain.

Fatigue is more common among people with depression, but many who are not depressed also have bothersome fatigue. Frequent tremor may also cause fatigue. Some people with Parkinson's note that their fatigue is different than the fatigue they experienced before the illness began. This and the fact that the fatigue responds to levodopa are arguments against depression as a major factor, and indicate that the best relief from fatigue will come with optimum adjustment of antiparkinson medication.

Sleep Problems

Up to two-thirds of people with Parkinson's sleep poorly. It's not clear whether the problem is related to the illness or to its treatment. Poor sleep is common as we get older—indeed, for some people it's a lifelong problem—but Parkinson's is associated with a whole new set of night-time problems. It's important that the patient, and perhaps the family as well, review the exact type of sleep upset with the physician; very worthwhile treatments are available.

More sleep upset occurs with more advanced Parkinson's, long-term use of levodopa, depression and cognitive problems. Bad dreams, muscle jerks, crying out and dyskinesias—all related to excess levodopa—may be major reasons for sleep disruption. Other problems associated with increased parkinsonism—pain, difficulty turning, frequent urination, cramps and muscle stiffness—need to be identified and treated.

A variety of defects in brain chemistry can also contribute to sleep upset. These include reduced dopamine, which creates motor problems, and serotonin deficiency, which causes depression and disrupts the sleep cycle. Specific sleep symptoms include insomnia, increased daytime sleepiness, upsets during sleep (including sleep violence), sleep benefit and morning worsening.

Insomnia

The common pattern for insomnia is wakening a few hours after falling asleep, being awake for a significant time, and wakening repeatedly after that. Nightmares may add to the problem. Insomnia is a frequent symptom of depression, and depression responds well to treatment, thus improving the insomnia.

Increased Daytime Sleepiness

People who sleep poorly at night are naturally likely to be fatigued and sleepy during the day. One of the major other causes can be medication. Anti-anxiety drugs taken at night or during the day will contribute to the problem. The more people take these medications, the worse the daytime sleepiness is likely to become. All the antiparkinson drugs can cause daytime sleepiness, but the dopamine agonists tend to be the worst offenders.

Upsets during Sleep

Upsetting dreams, and talking and/or walking during sleep, may all be signs that the dose of levodopa is about as high as the person can tolerate. Various muscle jerks that occur during sleep may also be related to levodopa. They do not usually awaken the person, but they can certainly disturb anyone sharing the bed. Tricyclic antidepressants may also increase night-time movements, and behavior upsets as well.

Sleep violence occurs in up to 15 percent of people being treated for Parkinson's. It may involve nocturnal kicking, running, punching, thrashing and pushing. Bed partners often report injury from these incidents. If the person with Parkinson's is wakened, he or she often complains of bad dreams.

Sleep Benefit

Up to 50 percent of people with Parkinson's say that they have improved motor function in the morning, and that they generally feel better then. They insist that this is their best time of day. The effect may last one to three hours, and it allows many people to delay their first dose of levodopa. Those who note this pattern tend to be older and male, and to have more night wakenings; they have usually had Parkinson's for a longer time. They do not report having more nightmares, hallucinations or sleep violence than people without sleep benefit.

Morning Worsening

Other people experience the opposite of sleep benefit; they feel worse on wakening. They usually keep their levodopa by the bed, to help them achieve mobility in the morning. A night dose of a dopamine agonist or long-acting levodopa preparation may help with this problem.

Pain and Sensory Symptoms

Normand was having difficulty getting out of bed in the morning. As he started to straighten his legs, his right foot would cramp. At first this had happened only once or twice a month, but now it was a problem almost every day.

Normand's doctor suggested that the cramping resulted from the low level of dopamine in Normand's brain at the start of the day. After a small adjustment to his Parkinson's medication, the cramping was reduced to a minor irritation.

Pain and other sensory symptoms are common among people with Parkinson's. The symptoms are variable and inconsistent, taking the form of cramping, numbness, burning, coldness or deep aching. The discomfort is usually more in the legs than in the arms—it's rarely in the face or neck—and it tends to be worse on the side of the body most affected by Parkinson's. There may also be abdominal pain. Pain is usually more proximal—in the upper ends of the limbs, toward the trunk—while numbness is more often in the fingers or toes.

The reason for these sensory effects is not clear, but they are frequently associated with dystonia (foot and toe cramping). Pain is often associated with motor fluctuations, and it is much more common among those who are depressed; it seems to be less frequent and less severe when people are experiencing an "on" period. Dystonia itself can cause painful spasms; these are usually in the foot and leg, but may also be in the neck, jaw, trunk, arm or hand. Neck or low back pain may be related to muscle rigidity or to spinal-disc disease.

Low back pain is common in the general population, and people with Parkinson's frequently have it, often as an initial symptom. They also tend to have headaches, which do not seem to be related to neck stiffness.

Internal Tremor

Internal tremor is a feeling of tremor inside the chest, abdomen, arms and legs, while no tremor is seen. It occurs in up to 40 percent of people with Parkinson's, and it's more frequent in those who also have other sensory symptoms such as aching, burning and tingling. The tremor is brief and episodic, is felt more on one side than on the other, and lasts five to thirty minutes. The tremor is felt more during "off" periods. The response to medication adjustments is not always good. Relaxation techniques, walking or simply changing the body position may help, and a mild tranquilizer clearly helps.

Internal tremor may precede the onset of Parkinson's; it can be a useful diagnostic factor to help screen people for Parkinson's before the diagnosis is clear.

Shoulder Pain

Shoulder-joint pain is a frequent problem in Parkinson's. Commonly called "frozen shoulder," it includes pain, a limited range of motion, and stiffness. It occurs because of decreased arm swing and shoulder movement. Frozen shoulder has been noted before the appearance of the main symptoms of Parkinson's, and it occurs on the side of the body first affected by the disorder. It is seen more in people with slowness and stiffness than in those with tremor.

Biceps tendonitis—tenderness of the biceps tendon over the front of the shoulder—may also cause shoulder pain. This condition may result from the posture that some people with parkinsonism develop, with the shoulders hunched forward. As well, the clavicle (collarbone) and shoulder are often injured in falls; these may result in very unpleasant chronic pain in the shoulder region.

Foot Pain
Foot pain and foot deformities are common in the older population generally. Many are caused by osteoarthritis. In addition, people may have arch problems, deviated or flexed toes, and corns and calluses.

Foot problems are often bothersome for people with Parkinson's, and some of the problems may be related to treatment. Leg pain, foot pain and flexing or extending of the toes may occur because of rigidity, or because prolonged levodopa treatment has led to extra involuntary foot movements. Foot cramps may cause the muscles of the foot to go into spasm, which positions the toes in a claw-like form. Foot problems related to dopamine levels in the brain respond to adjustments in the medication.

Dyskinesias triggered by levodopa sometimes cause abnormal foot and ankle movements when the person walks, which may contribute to imbalance and to the beginning of more persistent foot pain.

Ankle pain is less common, and it may be arthritic in origin, or related to foot problems. The person may need to be referred to a rheumatologist, for a definite diagnosis, before a treatment plan can be developed.

Falls

Falls are common among older people in the general population; of those over age sixty-five who live independently, 30 percent fall each year and 10 percent have a serious injury. Falls also result in loss of confidence, and people who fall often are more likely to be admitted to a nursing home.

Those suffering even mild problems of parkinsonism have a yet greater risk of falling. Falls may be caused by the loss of postural recovery reflexes. The tendency to fall may be further increased by parkinsonian slowness, poor vision and/or other medical problems, as well as many drugs. Falling may also result from low blood pressure that drops further when the person stands, causing fainting. Falls that result in hip fractures are becoming increasingly significant. Risk factors for serious falls include advanced age, poor nutrition, chronic medical problems, poor eyesight, osteoporosis (loss of bone mass), balance and gait disorders and muscle weakness. As people with Parkinson's have many of these risk factors, their risk of having a bad fall is that much higher.

Osteoporosis and Fractures

Betty's Parkinson's had been well controlled for over twelve years, but she had fallen several times during the past six months. Now she had had a particularly bad fall, trying to carry too much down a staircase. She found herself in the emergency room with a broken hip and a head full of questions. Would she ever be able to go back to living on her own? Why hadn't she asked for help with her parcels, or made two trips? Why hadn't she worn more practical shoes? What else could she have done to protect her bones?

Osteoporosis is thinning of the internal structure of the bones, which makes the bones break more easily. Almost everyone has some osteoporosis in later life, but people with Parkinson's

Facts about osteoporosis

Osteoporosis risk is higher in people who
- are female
- are older
- have had their ovaries removed and are not taking replacement hormones
- use oral steroids regularly
- went through menopause early
- have insufficient dietary calcium
- get little weight-bearing exercise
- drink excess alcohol
- smoke

have a higher incidence of osteoporosis than the general population of the same age. Also, loss of mobility—a common result of Parkinson's—increases the rate of bone loss. Since people with Parkinson's are more at risk of falling, and are more likely to have osteoporosis and the risk of serious fractures if they do fall, there are two steps they need to take: make every effort to prevent falls, and do as much as possible to prevent, diagnose and treat any osteoporosis.

Osteoporosis treatment is especially important for women, as they are more at risk of this condition—a woman aged fifty has a 15 percent risk of fracturing her hip in her remaining lifetime—but men get osteoporosis too. The loss of bone mass is diagnosed through a bone mineral density test—a simple, painless and widely available scanning procedure. The same test can be repeated from time to time to measure the response to therapy. The treatment of osteoporosis is complex and is changing rapidly these days; anyone who has this condition should have a treatment plan worked out by an endocrinologist (a specialist in treating hormone problems) or internist.

Bones can be strengthened by daily weight-bearing exercise, and by a diet high in calcium (1,200 to 1,500 mg per day).

The estrogen debate

Studies had long suggested that combined hormone replacement therapy (with estrogen and progesterone), given to women whose own hormone production had tapered off, helped lower heart-related health problems. Two recent, more precise studies have shown that, although hormone replacement helps prevent osteoporosis and decreases the risk of colon cancer, it increases the risk of strokes as well as breast and endometrial cancer. Since the balance of risk versus benefit varies from woman to woman, it is something a woman should discuss with her own doctor.

The best sources are milk, cheese and yogurt; two cups of milk daily provide 600 mg of calcium, plus vitamin D, which helps the body absorb calcium. Various calcium supplements are available in pill form; anyone with limited exposure to sunlight (which provides vitamin D) should be on supplemental vitamin D as well.

Estrogen therapy after menopause clearly reduces osteoporosis. It slows bone loss in the early postmenopausal years, the time when this loss would otherwise occur at its fastest rate.

A lifelong plan should be developed, using all the treatments outlined in varying combinations, to prevent osteoporosis in the early years, and to limit the condition once it develops.

Scoliosis

As Parkinson's progresses, people frequently develop a lean to one side, but in most cases this is quite minor. X-ray studies have shown that there are usually multiple spinal curves with an overall tilt to one side. We don't know why the spinal curvature occurs, but it is not usually due to underlying problems with the bones. In rare cases, specific problems have been diagnosed involving the muscles that run on either side of the spine. Sometimes the leaning becomes quite severe, impairing balance and leading to more falls. There is no relation between the side on which symptoms first appeared, and the side of leaning.

Leg Problems

Restless Leg Syndrome
Restless leg syndrome is an irresistible desire to move the legs or to walk. It is associated with numbness, aches and cramps, and also with delayed sleep onset and multiple wakenings. This condition is very common in Parkinson's but it's also seen in 10 percent of the general population. It can occur in the day but is normally markedly worse at night, just before sleep. A severe case is very upsetting, as it seriously disrupts sleep, resulting in sleep deficiency and daytime drowsiness. It can cause major problems in home, social and work life. A low red-blood-cell count and/or low iron body stores can contribute to an increase in restless leg symptoms. Anyone with this diagnosis needs to have his or her blood checked, as these problems can be easily reversed.

Leg Cramps
Leg cramps may affect people without Parkinson's, but they are a very frequent and upsetting problem in parkinsonism and, like restless leg syndrome, can cause major sleep disruption. The person is usually wakened by severe calf or foot pain, which is often prolonged. The pattern may vary over weeks and months. A number of other medical conditions may also cause cramps. These include low thyroid function, low potassium (usually related to the use of diuretics, or "water pills"), poor blood flow to the legs, and low-back disc disease with single or multiple nerve irritation. Blood-vessel problems and disc troubles are more likely to cause pain and cramps on walking. In people with Parkinson's, these cramps are usually a signal that the dopamine levels in the brain are low; a change of medication may help. However, the other possible causes listed above should also be considered.

Leg Swelling (Edema)
Lower-leg edema (swelling) is seen often in Parkinson's. If the swelling occurs in both legs, it may be a result of antiparkinson drugs, especially amantadine. Dopamine agonists also cause some leg swelling. Edema often occurs when there is a marked weight gain or a decrease in activity, such as that resulting from bradykinesia (slowness). It may also be a sign of kidney or heart failure (the latter is usually accompanied by shortness of breath). Discuss any such swelling with your doctor.

Digestive Problems
People with Parkinson's may develop significant, bothersome symptoms and problems involving a number of functions of the gastrointestinal (digestive) system. It has been shown that Lewy bodies, which are the typical marker of the Parkinson's process in the brain, are also seen in nerve cells of the digestive system. This means that the nerves associated with the digestive system are directly affected by the disease itself. Some symptoms are a nuisance; others are very serious, and may cause major problems that require careful attention.

Gastrointestinal problems include drooling, dry mouth, dental care problems, loss of smell and taste, swallowing difficulty, impaired gastric emptying, drug-related nausea and vomiting, constipation, poor nutrition and weight loss. Difficulty in swallowing is probably the most serious because it can lead to poor nutrition, and it increases the risk of accidentally breathing food into the lungs. Impaired stomach emptying can be serious because it results in poor absorption of medication.

Drooling
People with parkinsonism have normal production of saliva, but they often have difficulty and slowness in swallowing.

This, along with their tendency to adopt a lowered head position and to keep the mouth open, can cause excessive pooling of saliva. This leads to drooling, which is usually first a problem at night.

Dry Mouth

Dry mouth is a common side effect of both anticholinergic medications and tricyclic antidepressants. The dryness usually comes from a reduced flow of saliva, and is often most noticeable when the person is beginning new drug therapy. It tends to become less apparent as the body adjusts to the new therapy. Dry mouth may also be a result of breathing with the mouth open. Some people just have dry mouths naturally.

Dental Care Problems

People who have troublesome tremor or are slow in their everyday activities may neglect their teeth. Dental hygiene is important to health; poor dental care can cause infection, discomfort and difficulty in eating. Establish a good relationship with a dentist, and make regular visits.

Loss of Smell and Taste

It seems that people with Parkinson's have a decreased sense of smell, due to damage of the dopamine cells in the olfactory (smell) system. This loss can happen very early in the disease, and may be the first problem people notice. Because our senses of taste and smell are intimately connected, people who have diminished ability to smell may eat less, as they find less pleasure in food. This leads to poor nutrition and weight loss. Meals may be more tempting if extra attention is given to both the texture and the "eye appeal" of food. Increased use of spices, herbs and other flavorings can also help make up for someone's decreased sensitivity to taste.

Swallowing Difficulty

Swallowing difficulties (dysphagia) of some degree occur in up to 40 percent of people with Parkinson's, usually in later stages of the disease. If the problem is severe, it may limit the person's nutrition, and chest infections may result from food getting into the lungs (aspiration). Swallowing problems are usually more severe with solids than with liquids. Aging itself also causes the swallowing process to become less efficient.

There are various reasons why swallowing may be a problem. Some people have difficulty moving food around inside the mouth, or passing food to the back of the throat, because of a reduction in tongue movement. Some have trouble initiating the swallowing process. Some find that food or pills stick in the sides of the throat after the swallow is completed, causing coughing; this last symptom may be due to a weakness in the throat muscles that normally push the food through the throat and into the esophagus (food channel).

When swallowing is significantly impaired, people may also have associated respiratory symptoms, including coughing, choking, and shortness of breath at night. The clinic treatment team may assess the degree of swallowing difficulty by having the person swallow a few sips of water. Coughing and a wet hoarse voice in the minute after swallowing indicate a risk of lung problems (from food aspiration). This test can be helpful as an indication of a danger of aspiration, but more studies should be done to assess the person more thoroughly.

This degree of difficulty is uncommon; for most people, swallowing difficulties are a nuisance that can be controlled.

People are often reluctant to complain of swallowing problems unless the physician specifically asks about them. But swallowing problems have social implications; they can reduce the pleasure of eating, and make us uncomfortable eating in public. If swallowing difficulty is a symptom, the doctor should be told.

Impaired Gastric Emptying

Gastric emptying—the process of emptying the stomach—often works slowly in people with Parkinson's. The degree and timing of the problem are variable; it appears early in some people, even before treatment, while others never have much difficulty with it. The symptoms are a sensation of fullness, feeling satisfied almost immediately after eating, nausea, bloating, and discomfort after meals. Occasionally there may be vomiting.

Impaired gastric emptying may also reduce the effect of medication, as drugs have to pass through the stomach into the small intestine to be absorbed. If a dose of levodopa remains in the stomach, it may not take effect for as long as two hours—or it may not take effect at all. People with motor fluctuations have much more impaired stomach emptying, and this impairment may be one reason for the fluctuations.

Drug-Related Nausea and Vomiting

While impaired gastric emptying may cause nausea and vomiting in someone with Parkinson's, these symptoms are more often caused by medication used to treat the disease. Levodopa by itself can induce vomiting in most people. When it's combined with the drugs carbidopa or benserazide, vomiting and nausea decrease markedly and usually resolve with time. If nausea and vomiting develop during treatment, tests may be done to rule out causes not related to the Parkinson's.

Constipation

Constipation affects about 50 percent of those with Parkinson's; it's the most common gastrointestinal effect of the disorder. It's a source of much distress, as symptoms may include gas pain, abdominal distension (swelling from gas), hemorrhoids or, rarely, oozing of liquid stool. Factors contributing to constipation include the Parkinson's itself, which may affect

Factors contributing to constipation

- lack of daily exercise
- not enough bulk and fiber in the diet
- decreased muscle power generally
- limited fluid intake
- depression
- certain medications, including some antiparkinsonian drugs; for example, those with anticholinergic effect
- antacids
- diuretics ("water pills")
- certain anti-arthritis drugs, such as NSAIDs
- pain medications containing codeine

the nerve supply of the colon, causing stool to move slowly through the colon; insufficient intake of fluid and bulk; and general weakness and loss of muscle strength to push. People sometimes contribute to the problem by ignoring the urge to move their bowels.

There may also be abnormalities related to the rectum and anus, a problem that has been recognized only recently and is sometimes called pelvic-floor muscle dystonia. Instead of relaxing during a bowel movement, these muscles go into spasm, so that stool is not evacuated normally. Laxatives will not help this, but other medications can be helpful; see Chapter 6. If constipation is a problem, report this to the physician. Help is available.

Constipation may, rarely, be very severe, and may lead to obstruction of the bowel. The sudden onset of acute abdominal pain and marked abdominal distension in someone with severe chronic constipation suggests a twisted bowel (sigmoid volvulus), which requires emergency surgery.

Weight Loss and Poor Nutrition
There is no specific diet for most people with Parkinson's.

Diet and Parkinson's

Naturopaths and other practitioners of alternative medicine often pay great attention to the question of diet, and make many unusual recommendations. It is important to remember that, while some of these recommendations may seem plausible, none has been scientifically proven. The best advice is to eat a healthy balanced diet.

However, a good diet of at least three balanced meals per day, with a recommended balance (five to one) of carbohydrate and protein, is important.

If someone with Parkinson's is slowly losing weight, the disorder itself is usually a factor. Metabolism (energy-burning) is increased in Parkinson's, and the people with the most severely increased muscle tone and involuntary movements have the highest energy expenditure. It is suspected that there may also be a defect in their ability to process food to produce and store energy. In addition, people with Parkinson's may take in fewer calories due to taking too long to eat (and therefore not finishing meals); difficulty in cutting, chewing and swallowing food; reduced absorption from the digestive system; and poor dental health or poorly fitting dentures, which make chewing difficult.

As well, any infection will promote rapid weight loss. Depression, anxiety and memory loss may also be significant factors. All in all, weight loss and its possible causes should be carefully assessed.

Bladder Problems

Difficulties with urination are often part of Parkinson's. The first symptom is usually frequent urination at night (nocturia); often a sensation of incomplete bladder emptying is noticed. Also, a sense of urgency develops.

In most cases bladder dysfunction is mild, more a nuisance than a problem. However, for some people it's a major personal and social problem. Some need to urinate frequently during "off" periods, which may add to overnight problems. People typically use less medication at night, which results in more "off" time, which causes increased bladder frequency and more night-time wakenings. Some people, especially those with non-typical parkinsonism, have much more urinary difficulty; the urgency is overwhelming, the frequency is greater and incontinence of urine is common.

Drugs used in the treatment of Parkinson's may alter bladder function. Rare cases of bladder upset have been reported with levodopa or dopamine agonists. Drugs with anticholinergic activity tend to slow bladder function; rarely, they cause retention (inability to empty the bladder).

Because the bladder and the sexual organs have a similar nerve supply, bladder and sexual problems (see below) may occur in the same person.

Sexual Problems

Most sexual problems in Parkinson's are related to the illness itself. Sexual function decreases with age, and the loss of function can be up to six times faster in those with chronic illnesses such as Parkinson's.

Physical limitations such as tremor, slowness and reduced coordination add to the problem, especially since stiffness and tremor may increase with arousal and orgasm. Sexual dysfunction may be further aggravated by depression, which is also part of Parkinson's, and by anxiety and frustration as well. In men, the most common problem is difficulty in producing and maintaining an erection. In men and women alike, there is commonly a decrease both in interest in sexual activity, and in orgasmic function.

A reduction in libido (sex drive) has been noted even in young people with Parkinson's. Studies of sexuality in women with the disease show that many are dissatisfied with the quality of their sexual experience and with their partners. Many reported changed orgasms, with a number of high points and an abrupt stop without orgasm. Anxiety, inhibition, vaginal tightness and fear of incontinence are other factors that may inhibit sexual motivation.

Many drugs used for various conditions can decrease sexual function—common examples include codeine, thiazide diuretics, selective serotonin reuptake inhibitors and tricyclic antidepressants, allergy medication, cimetidine (stomach medication), drugs for anxiety, beta blockers (for tremor or hypertension) and certain monoamine oxidase inhibitors. Some of the new cardiac and antihypertensive (for high blood pressure) drugs also have adverse effects on sexual drive and function. Alcohol abuse and smoking also affect erectile function and contribute to impotence.

Intimacy and sexual expression are an important part of human relationships, and they are significant components of our quality of life. Sexual concerns should be discussed with the treatment team; these problems can often be treated. Don't be shy about asking for help; remember, these difficulties are part of the disease.

Postural Hypotension

Postural hypotension is a drop in blood pressure that occurs when someone changes position: rising from a chair, or getting out of bed. The effects of the low blood pressure may not be noticed until a few minutes after the change in position.

Blood pressure is controlled by the nervous system. When we change position, the blood flow is affected, and the body adjusts to ensure that the brain still receives enough blood (and therefore enough oxygen). But Parkinson's affects the nervous system, and it may disrupt this process of adjustment. Someone who changes position may feel lightheaded or faint, and may have momentary loss of vision; some people even lose consciousness and fall, perhaps suffering serious injury.

Postural hypotension can also cause unsteadiness in walking, which improves with treatment aimed at raising the blood pressure to a more normal level. This can make a significant improvement in quality of life.

Shortness of Breath

The air volume that someone inhales in one deep breath (vital capacity) is reduced in people with parkinsonism. This can lead to the sensation of being short of breath. Even less air will be inhaled in subsequent breaths, if the person struggles to take in more air. The problem tends to be worse in those who have greater disability from Parkinson's, and also in those who have motor fluctuations and dyskinesias.

This decrease in breathing is slowly progressive, and it's now being suggested that the problem should be treated as soon as it appears. If a program of exercise and chest physiotherapy is begun early, it may give long-term improvement in breathing function.

Skin Problems

People with Parkinson's commonly have problems with their skin, including oily facial skin, eyelid problems, dry body skin and sweating abnormalities.

Facial Skin

There may be excessive oil on the skin, especially around the scalp and face, resulting in dandruff, scaly skin and eyelid irritation. The oily skin is part of Parkinson's, and is more prominent in the central part of the face and the forehead, where sebaceous (sweat) glands are more numerous. This oiliness and scaliness is called seborrheic dermatitis and is usually easily controllable with proper skin care.

Eyelids
The eyelid irritation associated with oily facial skin is called blepharitis. The reduced blinking associated with Parkinson's also contributes to the irritation. If the irritation is severe, it may lead to inflammation of the corneas (the transparent fronts of the eyeballs).

Dry Body Skin
Although people with Parkinson's tend to have oily faces and hair, the rest of the body is usually very dry—a condition called xerosis. Therefore, products that are suitable for the face and hair may not be recommended for the body. The immobility of Parkinson's means that more prolonged pressure is applied to certain areas of the skin (most commonly on the buttocks), which can result in skin breakdown and open sores. Malnutrition, and irritation caused by excess perspiration or incontinence, can make this problem worse.

Sweating Abnormalities
Body temperature and sweating—used to bring down the temperature—are both controlled by the nervous system. Because Parkinson's affects the nervous system, the disease may lead to excessive sweating. It may also lead to impaired sweating, and abnormal sensations of heat and cold, or to abnormally low body temperature (hypothermia).

Excess sweating of the face and neck may result from being in a warm temperature, because the body's temperature-control system is impaired, but the problem can be made worse by exertion, fever or anxiety. Most sweating problems occur in people with more severe disability. Dopamine-replacement therapy tends to improve excessive sweating, at least in the early stages.

Not all excess sweating is caused by Parkinson's. Other possible causes—including large quantities of alcohol or ASA (aspirin), overactive thyroid gland, infection, menopause and certain tumors—should be ruled out.

Speech Problems (Dysarthria)
Speech is produced by air coming out of the lungs and crossing the vocal cords in the larynx (voice box). The larynx makes complex movements that set the air vibrating, and the lips, tongue and cheeks then shape the air into speech.

People with Parkinson's commonly experience problems with both speech and voice. However, not everyone has these difficulties, and those who do may have various problems to various degrees. The voice may become very weak, so it's difficult to hear. Sometimes the voice is strong enough at the beginning of a sentence but fades as the sentence progresses.

It's clear that breathing problems may reduce the volume of the speech. Recent studies have given us a better understanding of other aspects of this problem. Detailed electrical testing shows reduced activity in the muscles of the larynx, face and jaw, all of which contribute to the voice. In addition, reduced facial expression makes speech more difficult to understand. Direct observation of the larynx during speech shows reduced movement, and also tremor. Dopamine-replacement therapy may help the speech become louder, probably from better function of the face, lips and chest.

Even if dopamine-replacement therapy improves the low volume of the speech initially, the sound of the voice may remain monotone, lacking expression or intonation. Speech may lack clarity and precision due to difficulty in articulating clearly. The rate of speaking may be affected: phrases may come out in a rush, and it may be very difficult to slow the speech down. Some people find that they repeat sounds or words almost as though they are stuttering. There may be difficulty in beginning speaking, as well as inappropriate silences. Although many people manage quite well and don't consider their speech or voice problems to be too disruptive, some have greater impairment of speech and/or voice, which can significantly hamper their ability to communicate.

Some people develop word-finding difficulty, which is not necessarily related to memory impairment. For example, if you have difficulty generating simple words, your sentences will be broken up. If this occurs frequently, your speech will be hard to follow.

Handwriting

When Marco was in his late sixties, he began to notice that his handwriting was changing. The longer he wrote, the smaller his writing seemed to become. His wife asked if his arthritis was bothering him more, because she could hardly make out his notes.

Not long after that, Marco was diagnosed as having Parkinson's, and was put on medication. He soon found that it took him much less effort to write. His handwriting became larger and more readable, and his wife could once again read his messages.

Difficulty with handwriting is one of the very early Parkinson symptoms. The handwriting tends to become smaller as symptoms appear. (Writing that is very small and difficult to read is called micrographia.) Often, a doctor will ask for a handwriting sample, which can be used to make the diagnosis and/or assess the degree of the problem. Drug treatment for parkinsonian symptoms may improve the handwriting, but it seldom brings it back to normal.

Hand Deformity

Some people with longstanding, advanced disability develop hand deformities, although this seems to have happened less frequently in the past few years, with better drug therapy. Sometimes this problem results from chronic compression of the nerves in the upper arm, often because the person has been sitting in a poor position in a wheelchair. In this case the deformity appears as a bending of the wrist (wrist drop). This can be prevented with attention to bed and wheelchair position, and the use of padding and pillows. Other people develop severe flexion (curling) of the fingers into the palm, which causes chronic skin infection and makes the hand less functional. This problem may be improved by surgery to release tendons, so the hand can be straightened, but early use of splints and careful skin care will often avoid the need for surgery.

Visual and Eye Problems

Parkinson's does not cause loss of vision or blindness, but blurred vision and difficulty in reading, dry eyes and double vision are fairly common complaints of people whose illness is longstanding. Even early in the illness, before treatment, some people notice visual disturbances.

Our sharpness of vision depends on our ability to focus our eyes by slightly altering the shape of their lenses. When people have blurring of vision, especially when focusing or attempting to look at something up close, it's usually a side effect of some medication. However, even in early Parkinson's, difficulty reading (aside from the visual acuity problems normally treated by your eye specialist) are usually related to difficulty in focusing up close, and/or to dry eyes.

The most common drugs causing this are ones with anticholinergic effects, such as trihexyphenidyl, benztropine and tricyclic antidepressants. These drugs affect our ability to regulate the shape of the lenses, and this—plus the fact that our lenses grow more rigid as we age—causes the difficulty and blurring in near vision.

Occasionally, people have double vision and other visual symptoms during "off" spells, and these can be managed through a change in medication. Other visual problems—poor adjustment to low light levels, blurred vision, and spatial, color and pattern discrimination problems—are related to a lack of dopamine in the eyes' retinas and in the brain, and may respond to dopamine-replacement therapies.

When visual problems occur late in Parkinson's, they are more likely related to defects in the eye movements than to drug therapy. Parkinson's can cause subtle slowing of eye muscle movements, just as it slows muscles in other parts of the body. The eyes move with a jerky, ratchet-like movement that takes extra effort and causes eye-muscle fatigue. If this fatigue affects one eye more than the other, double or blurred vision results, because the two eyes are not moving in coordination.

Dry eyes are a frequent problem in healthy older people. Tears are normally spread across the eye by blinking, which we do unconsciously. Bradykinesia reduces the movements we do unconsciously. With less blinking the eyes become dry, and irritation, scratchiness or burning results. Drugs with anticholinergic effects also cause dry eyes.

FOUR

Managing the Symptoms of Parkinson's

Like other chronic disabilities, Parkinson's can be tough, depressing and demoralizing for everyone involved. The person with the disease will likely be struggling with self-image problems, as well as with the loss of independence in work and recreation, and with all the small nuisances that develop over the years of illness. Family members suffer the pain of watching a loved one cope with this loss, as well as the upset of seeing a parent or partner disabled, the feelings of inadequacy and guilt that may develop, and the changes they have to make in their own lives to look after the disabled person. To handle all this requires insight, a positive attitude and a unified effort by the patient, family, friends and treatment team.

When they are in public, people with Parkinson's are often concerned about what others may think of them. This and other elements of stress in social situations can increase their stiffness and tremor. With assistance such as counseling, stress management sessions and relaxation therapy, they can learn to handle the stress more effectively, and thereby reduce their symptoms. As well, the more thoroughly both they and their caregivers understand the disability and its complications, the more confident and capable they will feel in dealing with day-to-day trials. Parkinson's associations, support groups and exercise classes can be a great help by providing information, understanding, advice and positive feedback.

Various care programs are available, including respite (temporary relief) care both in and outside the home, in-home caregiver training, and adult daycare. Peer and group support are important; they reduce your stress and depression by allowing you to unburden yourself to others with the same worries: to exchange ideas, reduce your social isolation, share information on available resources, dispel any misconceptions you may have, and foster your self-confidence. There are also educational and counseling programs. These differ from support groups in that the focus is on teaching you skills such as problem-solving and coping tactics; it's easier to deal with new challenges if you are already prepared for them.

Studies show that people with chronic illnesses like Parkinson's often find that their "minor nuisances" are being ignored, although these nuisances may be having a major effect on their quality of life. The problems in question vary, depending on the person and the stage of the illness. They range from being unable to get an arm into a jacket sleeve, to being constipated, to being wakened frequently in the early morning by cramping feet. Fortunately, the tendency of caregivers to underestimate lesser problems is now beginning to change, and quality of life is now a major focus of many care programs. Treatments to improve the physical and mental state of the patient will raise the caregiver's quality of life as well. Scales have been developed to measure the quality of life of both the patient and the caregiver, and are now being incorporated into research studies, to ensure that treatments are not just improving a symptom but also having an impact on quality of life.

Studies also show that treating a patient's depression and mobility problems will give the caregiver great relief. Of course, the stress and depression of the caregiver increase as the patient worsens; a depressed patient with memory loss is much more of a burden than someone who has only mobility problems. On top of that, caregivers often have their own health problems and physical limitations. If the medical team keeps assessing the quality of life of both the patient and the caregiver, problems can be identified early, and appropriate steps can be taken to relieve the situation.

Both patients and caregivers (including physicians and nurses) should be careful that the lesser "nuisance problems" of Parkinson's are attended to; they are too easily overlooked. Something positive and helpful should come out of every physician or clinic visit; a "doing something" approach can be a great comfort and morale booster for the patient. Patients will do better, and be more comfortable with their illness, if they have hope.

Keeping a Positive Outlook

Whether you have Parkinson's yourself, or you are caring for someone who does, it's very important to remain as cheerful and optimistic as you can. Don't dwell on the long-term outlook of the illness; take one day at a time. Don't let the illness stand between you and other people. Remember that the close feelings and positive aspects of a relationship with a partner tend to start decreasing early in the illness; work on maintaining your bond.

Tips for the Person with Parkinson's

- Educate yourself; learn as much as possible about your disability and its likely progression, and about treatment and research.
- Try to stay as independent as possible.

- Focus on the improvements you get, whether they are small or large, and make the most of them.
- Thank those who are looking after you, frequently. They aren't having much fun either, and your thanks will help them cope.
- Find out whether physiotherapy and/or speech therapy can help you adapt to, and improve, certain aspects of your disability.
- Learn to delegate your responsibilities if you are unable to fulfill them, or if you find them frustrating.
- Remain active; exercise will help you maintain your level of function. Your body will tell you if it's time to switch to a less strenuous activity.
- Pace yourself. Set aside time for daily rest periods if you are tiring more easily.
- Keep up your social life, even if it becomes more limited or if you have to choose different activities.
- Try to overcome feelings of embarrassment when you are with others or in public. Admit to having Parkinson's; people will respond to your own secure self-image. Remember that many healthy people are very uncomfortable with illness. Your attitude can influence them.
- Mention any small nuisances that are bothering you, and seek help in dealing with them.

Tips for the Caregiver
- Try to keep life as normal and active as possible, but recognize that Parkinson's slows people down; you may have to adjust your living style to allow the disabled person enough time to complete activities.
- Recognize that the disabled person's problems are real, even if they change from hour to hour. The frequent changes are part of Parkinson's and its drug treatment.

- Put yourself in the other person's position for a better understanding of how he or she feels.
- Accept the fact that poor memory and confusion can be part of Parkinson's, and are made worse by many drugs. Discuss these problems with the treatment team; they may be able to improve matters.
- Recognize that past emotional problems and anxieties— of the patient and/or caregiver—may become worse.
- Counseling and emotional care are available; ask for them if you need them.
- Understand that 40 percent of people with Parkinson's suffer from depression.
- Don't forget to say "You look great" or "You look better today"; such encouragement is especially inspiring and reassuring when it comes from someone close.
- Accept the fact that the person may deny having the illness, or may downplay its severity; denial is a common method of adjusting to Parkinson's.
- Try to get ongoing help in the home, and to have your loved one spend some time in respite care. You will be more able to cope if you've had some relief. Dealing with Parkinson's is a job; sometimes you need a holiday.
- Keep some time for yourself. Develop outside interests and hobbies.
- Plan time together on a mutual activity you both enjoy, like the theater or walks.
- Accompany the person to medical and other appointments, so that you can gain information, express your concerns and make treatment suggestions. However, don't speak for the other person, if he or she is able to communicate without your intervention.

Assistive Devices

Helen was starting to have serious difficulty getting dressed. She needed more and more help from her spouse, and her loss of independence was upsetting her. She wondered if there was anything she could use to help her cope better on her own. When she thought the problem through, she realized that by keeping a chair close to the closet so that she could sit down when she needed to, and by choosing appropriate clothes and shoes, she could make dressing much easier. Then she did some research, and discovered that she could buy long-handled tongs to reach for things, and a long-handled shoehorn. Pretty soon she was dressing independently again.

In the course of their daily activities, people with Parkinson's may encounter a variety of practical difficulties. Many *assistive* devices and techniques have been developed to get past these obstacles. Your physician may refer you to an occupational therapist who can suggest safety measure you can take (such as adding handrails), teach you how to use assistive devices such as reaching tongs and dressing sticks, and show you how to conserve your energy and time. Support agencies are also familiar with this equipment; they can advise you on where to buy and how to use it. Most items that aren't in the general marketplace are readily available from medical and health supply stores, and there may even be government or insurance programs to help cover the cost.

In addition, you may be able to come up with simple, inexpensive solutions of your own, through the imaginative use of normal household implements, supplemented by a little ingenuity and perhaps a hammer and saw. If a few assistive devices, purchased or homemade, can help you maintain your independence, they may be well worth the investment of time and money.

Here are some suggestions about particular areas of daily living.

For Dressing
- If buttoning shirts and pants is a problem, use Velcro fasteners and zippers. Just remove the old buttons and replace them with Velcro strips.
- Replace regular shoelaces with elastic ones that have loops at both ends. Instead of tying your shoes, you slip one loop of the elastic over the other and twist. To take your shoe off you just untwist the loops. Alternately, choose shoes with Velcro straps.
- Wear track suits or pants with elastic waists to make dressing more comfortable and simpler.
- Have thumb-pulls sewn into pants and underpants so they are easier to pull on and off.
- Use a dressing stick or a cane to pull up pants and underwear.
- To pull on or slip on shoes, use a long shoehorn or long-handled reaching tongs.
- Have a sturdy chair in the area where you get dressed, preferably close to the shower.

In the Bathroom
- Use an elevated toilet seat.
- Install safety grab bars close to the toilet seat.
- Install handrails or grab bars for the bathtub and shower, and use non-slip mats.
- Hang an easy-to-open knapsack on a hook mounted low and close to the toilet, where personal toiletries will be handy.
- Consider buying one of the special chairs designed for use in the bathtub or shower.

- If it's a problem to stand or bend over in the shower or bath, install a shower hose.
- Consider replacing the bathtub with a shower, so you don't have to step over the high edge of the bathtub.
- Consider installing one-handled levers on taps, instead of knobs. Faucets with infrared sensors are also available for home use, but are quite expensive.
- Keep a long-handled brush or sponge for washing below the knees.
- Use a wash mitt or terrycloth glove instead of a washcloth.
- Put foam rubber grips on the handles of toothbrushes and other tools, to hold them more securely.
- Rather than fighting a slippery bar of soap, buy the kind that comes on a rope, or use liquid soap from a dispenser bottle.
- Remember that electric razors and toothbrushes may be easier to use effectively.
- Full-body dryers are available, for people who have difficulty managing towels.

In the Bedroom

- Try satin sheets; they allow easier movement in bed.
- Elevate the bed on wooden blocks to make it easier to get in and out of bed. Make sure the blocks are securely placed.
- Attach a bed rope to the foot of the bed, with knots tied along its length; this makes it easier to pull yourself up in bed. (The rope must be long enough to reach your chest when you're lying down.)
- Have a floor-to-ceiling grab bar installed beside the bed to help you pull yourself up. Alternately, there are grab bars designed to slide partly under the edge of the mattress, with the rest of the bar up the side of the bed.

- Keep your cane or walker near your bed at night; keep a flashlight as well, or have adequate nightlights.
- Consider getting a bedside urinal or commode (chair with bedpan) to avoid night-time trips to the bathroom.

For Eating

- Use a clip-on ring designed to provide an edge for the plate. This prevents food being pushed off the plate.
- Use a rocker knife for cutting with one hand. The tip of the knife is designed so that it can also be used as a fork.
- Use a combination spoon/fork, so that you don't have to switch utensils for the different food items on the plate.
- Serve hot fluids in an insulated drinking cup with a drinking spout in the cover, to prevent spills and keep the drinks warm longer.
- Have your plate on a warming tray during dinner, to keep food hot while you eat.

For Homemaking

- Use "extend-your-reach" handles on mops and other tools, and a long-handled dust pan, for dusting and cleaning up spills.
- Buy aprons with large pockets to keep hands free to hold onto a walker or cane.
- Install a spray hose attachment to the kitchen tap for rinsing dishes and vegetables.
- Keep a lazy Susan (turntable tray) on the kitchen counter to store supplies within easy reach.
- Replace knob-operated taps for your garden hose with lever taps that have a 90-degree rotation between the "on" and "off" positions. Replace outside hose connections with snap-on, snap-off connectors.

For Writing

- For handwriting, buy rubber grips for pens and pencils so they will be easier to grasp; you'll find these at medical, stationery or school supply stores. Felt pens may also be helpful.
- If you don't know how to use a computer, consider learning. Computers are available quite cheaply now, and word-processing programs are simple to use. While keyboarding may sound laborious, a computer lets you reuse blocks of writing (shopping lists, or names and addresses, for example) indefinitely. Perhaps you have a child (or grandchild!) who can help you get started.
- If you have difficulty writing, voice recognition software has greatly improved. Once you "teach" the computer to recognize your speech, you talk into a microphone and the computer types out your words.

Gait

Gait (walking) problems are a major and serious component of the slowness (bradykinesia) of Parkinson's. They can contribute greatly to a decline in general health, since keeping active and fit improves general health, avoids a multitude of serious problems and prolongs life. For all of these reasons, people with Parkinson's, and their family and their health care team, should make every effort to promote mobility and exercise.

Tom had been staying active and enjoying his regular exercise program, which included walking to the local mall. Now, however, he found that his feet would suddenly stop moving as he approached the escalator. He also noticed that his feet seemed to "stick to the floor" when he went to get food out of his pantry at home. He reported this to his doctor, who adjusted his dose of levodopa. Tom's walking problems didn't disappear, but they did improve.

"Freezing" is a major problem that can be very difficult to treat, and may not respond to standard antiparkinson therapy. When someone freezes, it's as if the feet are stuck to the floor; the problem lasts from seconds to a minute, and may also affect speech, writing and manual chores such as toothbrushing. Freezing is more common and severe in atypical parkinsonism, including progressive supranuclear palsy, vascular parkinsonism and hydrocephalus, and in these disorders it responds less well to the tricks that can be effective in classic Parkinson's (see below).

Freezing may occur when movement is begun or when it is changed. Four types have been identified:

- sudden temporary freezing while walking
- "start hesitation" such as rising from a chair and then being unable to step forward
- "turning hesitation" when trying to change direction
- "terminal hesitation," being unable to complete a final action such as sitting down or stepping up onto a weigh scale

Many freezing periods happen when someone is distracted or interrupted during a movement. Drug treatment for freezing may not be very effective, but adjusting the dosages of levodopa and dopamine agonists is worth trying.

In another gait problem, *festination*, the person leans forward, takes short steps, begins to almost run and frequently falls. This is more likely to happen to people who are not on medication, and medication usually clears it up.

Tips for Initiating Movement and Walking
If you are having gait problems, the following suggestions may help. Read the whole list over, and try various "tricks" over a few days; see which ones work for you, and incorporate them into your daily routine. Note that many of these tricks involve motor and sensory cues, and depend on you paying close attention to the action you want to initiate.

- Use a marching rhythm to move. There are a number of ways to do this. Wear a portable tape or CD player with a headset, and play marching music and swing your arms; or count rhythmically, or sing a marching song. If you use a cane, tap the floor to a regular beat, then walk to the beat. If not, tap your hip with your hand. Any strong, rhythmical pattern will help.
- If you use a walker, it should have wheels and brakes. This helps you walk more smoothly and without interruption.
- Alter your weight distribution and your direction of movement. If you can't go forward, step backwards or sideways. Push down on your foot before lifting it, or lift up your toes and shift your weight to the back of your heels. Stamp your feet, or rock from side to side, or bend your knees and then straighten up. Raise your arms in a sudden short motion or clap your hands.
- If you are "frozen" and you use a cane, place it in front of your foot and try to kick it. Or use an upside-down walking stick (a cane with a straight-edged handle at the bottom instead of the top); place this in front of your foot, close to your toes, and then step over it.
- Minimize distractions and interruptions if freezing is a problem.

- Use concentration strategies such as watching other people walk, or picturing white lines on the floor to step over, or else focus your attention on taking long steps.
- A laser pointer directed a few inches in front of your foot can provide a visual cue to initiate walking, as you think of stepping either on or over the beam.

Here are some additional tips to improve a slow, shuffling gait that causes tripping.

- Walk with a wide stance, lifting your foot forward and placing the heel down first. Make sure that your head is up and your shoulders are back. Look ahead instead of down, and swing your arms.
- Turn by walking in a circle, using your hands for guidance. Don't cross one foot in front of the other, and don't have your weight on the pivoting foot, or your feet will get tangled.
- Use a cane if necessary, but be sure it's the right height. To determine the correct cane height, put your hands by your side and stand straight; the head of the cane should be level with your wrist. The cane should have a rubber tip and, in winter, an ice pick. If you must grip the cane tightly for prolonged periods, the tendons in your palm may be injured, resulting in painful stiff fingers. Wrapping the handle with a soft, spongy material will help.
- Use a walker if necessary. Check with your doctor, nurse or physiotherapist for the one best suited to your needs. Some people do very well with wheeled walkers, and excellent, safe models are available. Wheeled walkers are preferable for people with Parkinson's because of their difficulties with gait initiation and freezing. Some even have seats and baskets. U-shaped bases give improved stability. Walkers give a real boost to confidence and inde-

pendence. Some people are reluctant to try a walker, but most are pleasantly surprised at their new freedom. Ask if your clinic has one you can try out.

- Plan a simple daily routine of exercises to maintain muscle tone and coordination (see "Home Exercise Program," later in this chapter).
- Have your physician refer you to a physiotherapist or rehabilitation specialist for gait training and the proper use and choice of a cane or walker.
- If you tire after walking a long distance, take along a walker with a seat, or bring a wheelchair to rest in.
- If you move too slowly, review all your medications— especially any recent changes—with your physician. An increase in levodopa, and the addition of amantadine, or a dopamine agonist, may improve your speed.

If you find that you are moving too quickly (festination, see above), stop and start again slowly.

Tips for Rising from a Chair or Bed

People with bradykinesia (slowness of movement) often find it difficult to get up from a chair, couch or bed. In fact, the ability to rise from a firm medium-height chair, without using your hands to push yourself up, is one of the best measures of the degree of slowness. This slowness typically responds well to dopamine-replacement therapies.

For chairs:

- Move to the front edge of the chair, then lean forward and place your feet widely, firmly on the floor under your body. Use your hands, on either the arm or the seat of the chair, to push yourself up into a standing position. It may help to use a rocking motion, or to count to three.

- Ask your physiotherapist about exercises to increase the strength of the muscles involved.
- Ask your doctor if your medication should be adjusted; extra levodopa may help.
- Avoid low and soft-cushioned chairs. Choose a chair with armrests when possible.
- Put small blocks, about two inches (5 cm) high, under the rear legs of your chair, for a slight forward tilt. You can buy blocks specially made for this; consult your occupational therapist for more details. Make sure the blocks are not high enough to make the chair unsteady!
- Try an adjustable-height office chair (with armrests), or one of the "self-rising" chairs with a motorized seat that slowly rises and tilts you toward a standing position.

For beds: in addition to the tips mentioned earlier in this chapter,

- When you sit down on the bed, place yourself at the right distance from the head of the bed, so that when you lie down you are already in the position for sleeping.
- To turn over in bed, lie flat on your back, bend your knees, put your arms across your chest and turn your head to the side you want to turn to. Then let your legs fall to that side, and your body will follow. Even if you are quite disabled and have poor balance, proper medication will probably allow you to turn in bed.
- To get out of bed, turn onto your side and support yourself on your elbow and forearm while gripping the edge of the bed with your hands. Bend your knees up toward your chest and place your toes near the edge of the bed. As you swing your feet down to the floor, push yourself up into a sitting position, first with your elbow, then with your hands. Sit on the side of the bed long enough to let

your blood pressure stabilize, so you don't get dizzy and perhaps fall.

Tips for the Family

- Offer to help with a light touch to the arm or shoulder. **Do not push or pull.**
- Step in front and ask the person to mimic your actions. Say, "Follow me," and walk ahead.
- Minimize distractions and avoid interruptions when walking with the person. For example, instead of stopping in the doorway and turning to meet the person, walk right into the room.
- Ask the person what distractions are most likely to cause freezing.
- Provide obstacles for the person to step over, such as your foot, or pieces of paper spaced on the floor, to be used as visual cues to start the movement. If the person "gets stuck" (frozen), try raising his or her leg slightly.
- Use simple verbal commands, such as "Lift right foot!", "March, left-right, left-right!" or "Swing your arms!"
- Remind the person frequently about the concentration strategies discussed above.

Memory Loss

Memory loss can be very frustrating. You'll have less trouble with it if you remember two basic rules.

First, make a special effort to create a memory in the first place. When you hear a word or name you don't want to forget, repeat it several times to familiarize yourself with the sound. When you are told something you want to remember, connect the word to something meaningful to you. Usually a visual image is effective. For example, if you're meeting your son at the Parrot Restaurant, imagine him with a large parrot on his shoulder!

Secondly, **be relaxed**. The less tense you feel, the more open your mind is to new information, and the easier it is to recall old information. If you can't recall a name or fact, relax and wait; there's a good chance that it will come back to you in a short time.

Here are some other tips to help compensate for memory loss.

- Avoid demanding and stressful situations whenever possible, especially ones where you have to make decisions rapidly. Allow yourself time to listen to people; ask them to address you one at a time, so you don't have to keep up with everyone at once. With a little time, you'll get there just as well.
- Develop routines; if you always put something in a certain place, you should always be able to find it.
- Carry a notebook; write down important items and date them. This is much more practical than carrying multiple scraps of paper with notes jotted on them.
- Use a large calendar to keep track of important events and appointments. Place the calendar where it will be most handy—perhaps by the phone, or in the kitchen.
- Handheld electronic organizers are easy to operate and are becoming more and more sophisticated. You can use one to make notes and keep a calendar and address book, and newer versions even have voice recorders.

Confusion and Hallucinations

Confusion and hallucinations are almost always a side effect of medication; the first measure against them is to consult the physician about adjustments to the drug schedule. As well, be sure the person is eating and drinking well. If the hallucinations are mild, explain to the person that the things being seen (bugs are common) are not really there, and that the problem is caused by the medication. Most people soon learn to recognize what is real and what isn't. Here are some other tips that may help.

- Most mild illusions occur at night, when shadows are misinterpreted as animals or people. Turn on more lights to reduce the shadows.
- Also turn on the lights when the person wakes after a vivid dream or nightmare, to make it easier to focus on reality.
- Some hallucinations and illusions are persistent, but mild and not upsetting. Despite reassurance, the person insists that what's being "seen" is real. Rather than causing constant friction, it may be better to avoid arguing about it.
- Someone who is having hallucinations is likely to do better in a familiar environment; being moved out of it into a hospital, new residence or relative's home may increase the problem.
- In rare cases, hallucinations are extreme and are accompanied by delusions and paranoia. The person may become agitated, aggressive or violent. In a case like this, don't provoke a confrontation; do what you can to prevent injury. Call for medical assistance—even 911— if necessary. Don't panic; a change in medication will decrease these alarming symptoms.

Emotional Problems

Depression
Depression is common among people with Parkinson's, but it's also very treatable. Everyone involved should be on the watch for this problem, and should be prepared to treat it optimistically. Keep in mind, however, that people with Parkinson's often show a lack of facial expression, which does not necessarily

mean sadness or depression; the person may be very interested in, or amused by, whatever's going on.

We do not know for certain the reason behind this increased incidence of depression, but it is likely that a number of factors are involved. Chronic diseases are generally associated with a higher rate of depression. As well, people with Parkinson's are at an age when they may be dealing with additional stressful issues, such as retirement, downsizing of the family home, or loss of a spouse or family member. There is also an increased incidence of thyroid problems in people with Parkinson's. Thyroid problems can cause depression, and they share some features of Parkinson's, but they can be easily diagnosed and treated. If someone is depressed and has Parkinson's, the possibility of thyroid problems should be considered.

However, most depression in Parkinson's is thought to be related to the neurochemical losses occurring within the brain. There is evidence that the loss of dopamine can be a factor, but the loss of other neurochemicals (serotonin, norepinephrine) is thought to play a larger role. We now have many different classes of medications that act on a variety of these non-dopamine neurochemicals, which are very effective in people with Parkinson's and depression. In general, these medications are also very well tolerated.

The first step in treatment is identifying any life stresses that may be contributing to the depression. A long-term plan must then be worked out to minimize the stress and improve the quality of life. A daily exercise and stretching routine is highly recommended. Motor symptoms of the Parkinson's should be treated as effectively as possible. If these steps do not relieve the depression, specific antidepression drug treatment can be started.

Selective serotonin reuptake inhibitors (SSRIs) and tricyclic antidepressants have been the mainstay of depression therapy in Parkinson's. There are two common types of depression: *apathetic* (withdrawn) and *agitated*. SSRIs are used for people who are apathetic, as they have an activating effect. The more common SSRIs used are fluvoxamine, paroxetine and sertraline.

Tricyclic antidepressants are used for people who are agitated, as they have sedative effects. They do not worsen Parkinson's, but because they have anticholinergic effects they are more likely to induce delirium, especially in those who are memory-impaired. They may also aggravate low blood pressure problems. Desipramine and nortriptyline tend to be tolerated best.

Other antidepressants that work in different ways but also play a role in treating Parkinson's depression include venlafaxine, nafazodone, buproprion and trazadone. Each has advantages as well as disadvantages. If you try one antidepressant, and it doesn't work or you experience side effects, it is important to discuss this with your doctor; there are many others to choose from.

Drug treatment of Parkinson's patients with depression usually lasts at least six to eight months; often it is long-term.

Agitation, Anxiety and Panic Attacks

These problems can be managed with short-acting minor tranquilizers and may also require adjustments to the regimen of antiparkinson drugs; consult your physician.

Fatigue

Studies of people with Parkinson's make it clear that dopamine-replacement medications can significantly reduce fatigue. The side of the body most affected by the Parkinson's will improve the most. A new medication called modafinil has been shown to be helpful for some individuals who have Parkinson's with profound fatigue and drowsiness.

When fatigue is an issue, accept the fact that everyday activities require more time and increased effort to complete, and plan the day carefully. Pace the schedule; allow time to complete each activity, and include rest periods. Plan special activities for the time of day when medications are most effective. Make use of the many products already mentioned that reduce the effort of routine activities.

It may also be worth trying an exercise program to improve muscle conditioning, since people with Parkinson's tend to have problems using oxygen efficiently. Ask your doctor or physiotherapist about this.

Sleep Problems

If insomnia is a problem, the whole pattern of sleep should be reviewed with the physician. It's important to identify any Parkinson's-related factors that may be involved, such as muscle stiffness or cramping, nightmares, memory loss or depression. (Insomnia and daytime sleepiness are frequently symptoms of depression, and in that case they usually respond well to treatment for the depression.)

If the underlying problem is anxiety or a transient life upset, your doctor may prescribe a short-acting minor tranquilizer for a brief while, until the upsetting situation can be resolved.

Increased daytime sleepiness may also be related to the antiparkinson drugs, in which case an adjustment may help.

Here are some things you can do yourself to combat insomnia and daytime sleepiness. For drug therapies see Chapter 6.

Tips for Insomnia
- During the day, be more socially active. Get plenty of bright light, and try not to spend a lot of time in bed.
- Exercise regularly, but not right before going to bed.
- Daytime naps are fine, especially if your overnight sleep

is poor; as your sleep improves, try to make them shorter. Naps should not be too late in the day, however, or they will interfere with your ability to fall asleep.
- Avoid caffeine and alcohol in the evening.
- Avoid eating a large meal before going to bed.
- Drink warm milk before bedtime.
- Don't go to bed too early. Establish a regular schedule of going to bed and getting up. Set your alarm clock for a certain time every morning, and get up at that time no matter how much sleep you've had. A consistent routine establishes a sleep cycle for your body.
- Develop a bedtime ritual, as it will remind your body that it's time to go to sleep. Take a warm bath and perhaps read part of a good book before sleeping.
- Before going to bed, try to ensure that you are relaxed and tired. Being generally stressed, or worried about how much sleep you are about to get, will only keep you awake.
- Learn relaxation exercises and use them as you settle yourself for sleep.
- If you are still unable to sleep after being in bed for some time, get up and read or watch television for a while. Trying to force yourself to sleep only wakens you further.

Tips for Daytime Sleepiness
- Increase your caffeine intake.
- Try to become more active—if not physically, then mentally. Daytime sleepiness may result from boredom and lack of social activities.
- Plan a regular routine of exercise, about five to ten minutes two or three times daily.
- If you feel depressed, seek medical advice.
- Ask your doctor whether some other medical problem, such as low thyroid function, may be a factor.

Pain and Sensory Symptoms

People with Parkinson's may experience sensory symptoms, including pain—occasionally quite severe pain—that are associated with the disorder. These pains and sensory symptoms may appear before the Parkinson's is diagnosed, and they may clear when medication is started. For details of the drugs used in Parkinson's, see Chapter 6.

Before pain is blamed on the Parkinson's, however, other possible causes should be considered. Arthritis may cause painful hip or shoulder bursitis, for example, and diabetes and vascular disease may cause pain in the feet. Always keep your doctor informed of any new or persisting pain.

Once other medical conditions have been ruled out, it may be possible to relieve the discomfort through a number of non-drug strategies, such as heat, massage or increased activity. Even simply elevating the affected limb may reduce the pain. Discuss these approaches with your physician.

Lower back pain sometimes begins early in Parkinson's; it may clear with drug therapy but later return as the illness worsens. Physiotherapy may help. In some cases lower-spine disc surgery may be the only answer.

"Frozen" shoulder often improves with antiparkinson therapies. Range-of-motion exercises and moving the shoulder with heat (in a warm shower) may also help significantly, as may non-prescription anti-inflammatory drugs such as ASA (aspirin) or ibuprofen. (Discuss these with your doctor first.) If shoulder pain becomes severe and persistent, ask to be referred to a physiotherapist or rheumatologist.

Tips for Dealing with Pain
- A program of regular, gentle exercise may reduce the pain or discomfort caused by stiff joints and muscles, and stooped posture.

- Specially designed cushions that relieve neck or back pain are available in health supply stores. Ask a physiotherapist or occupational therapist to aid you in making the right choice.
- Relaxation therapies of various kinds may be helpful. Check with your doctor before trying them.

Falls

As mentioned earlier, falling is a common hazard for people with Parkinson's. Difficulties such as muscle weakness, balance problems, poor vision and other factors unrelated to the disorder may increase the risk. All too often, falls result in broken bones, which can lead to more depression, and further undermine the person's health. Yet with care and forethought most falls can be prevented.

You are more likely to fall if you wear the wrong shoes or slippers. Be sure your footwear fits well and gives good support. Wear leather-soled shoes; rubber or crepe soles grip the floor, making it more difficult to walk, especially with a toe-first gait. Keep your shoes in good repair. For icy weather strap "ice grips" onto your shoes or overshoes; you'll find them in health supply stores. Women should, of course, avoid high heels.

Medication is another major risk factor. Various drugs for a wide variety of medical problems can increase your risk of falling. Sleeping medication, long-acting tranquilizers, drugs for blood pressure and antidepressants often contribute to falls. If you have had a fall or a near-fall, ask your doctor to review all your medications. He or she may also want to do a neurological exam, checking for other possible reasons, such as muscle weakness, nerve disease, inner-ear disease, problems of the cerebellar (balance) system and signs of stroke.

Have your eyes checked; maybe you need new glasses or cataract surgery. Be sure you're following a proper diet; malnutrition significantly increases the chance of falling, as it can lead to muscle and nerve problems. Hip and knee arthritis and foot problems are other possible reasons for falling.

Sudden falls with a loss of consciousness are usually related to an irregular heart rhythm or to postural hypotension (low blood pressure on standing). Your heart rhythm can be checked with a heart monitor that you wear for a period of twenty-four hours or more. If your falls seem to result from postural hypotension, have your blood pressure checked in different positions—lying down, sitting and standing. Ongoing low blood pressure can also cause chronic unsteadiness in walking, which is often overlooked.

Preventing Falls and Injuries around the House
- Ensure adequate lighting, especially at the top and bottom of stairs and in dark hallways. Use nightlights.
- Remove loose scatter rugs. Consider wall-to-wall carpeting; it will soften a fall and possibly prevent broken bones.
- Don't leave shoes, clothing and other objects on the floor.
- Remove furniture from traffic areas. Remove door sills too, if possible.
- Pets like cats and dogs may not be advisable, as they can trip you.
- Make sure furniture and appliances are stable.
- Install handrails on staircases.
- If you use a cane or walker, keep it near your bed at night.
- Maintain outdoor steps and walks in good repair. Be aware of any slippery surfaces and try to avoid them; correct them if possible.
- A plastic bag fastened on the car seat will make entering and exiting the car much easier.
- Don't wax bare floors. Wipe up spills immediately.
- Install a telephone on each level of the house, or have a portable phone. Use an answering machine and set it to

answer after the fourth or fifth ring, so you won't feel you have to rush to the phone.

- Have your physician refer you to an occupational therapist for a home safety assessment, and expert suggestions. For example, normal beds and toilets tend to be too low; safety rails, a raised toilet seat or a commode chair fitted over the toilet may be helpful. Bed rails are a wise safeguard for someone who has confusion, hallucinations or vivid dreams. A seat belt on a wheelchair will keep a confused, unstable person from getting up unassisted.
- Have your physician refer you to a physiotherapist for an assessment, walking advice and tips about proper choice and use of a cane or walker.

In the Bath

- Have someone with you when you bathe if you have a history of falling or unsteadiness.
- Avoid bath products that leave the tub slippery. Use non-slip bathtub and floor mats.
- Use bathtub aids such as a bath bench, table and handrails (see "Assistive Devices," earlier in this chapter).
- Sit down when dressing or undressing.
- Don't lock the bathroom door. Be sure someone is within hearing distance while you're bathing.

Getting Help

Remember the saying "Hope for the best, but plan for the worst." Consider the places you might possibly fall, and ask yourself how you would get help. This is especially important if you live alone.

- Arrange a daily contact with a friend or relative.
- Wear a whistle, if help is within hearing range.

- Keep a telephone or alarm where you can reach it from the floor.
- Consider a personal alarm system. This kind of alarm can be linked to your telephone or your existing home security system, or it can function separately. You simply wear a button around your neck or wrist and press it if you're in trouble. The monitoring company then tries calling you; if you say you need assistance, or you don't answer, they send help. Contact your local Parkinson's association, your telephone company or a home security company for more information.

Recovering from a Fall

Suppose you are on the floor on your back, and there is no one to help you. Use a rocking motion to turn onto your side. Now use your hands to push yourself up to a sitting position. Turn slowly and come onto all fours, and crawl to a chair or a heavy piece of furniture. Bring up your hands, spaced apart, on either side of the chair. Bring one knee up so your best leg is forward; use your hands to press down on the chair and then push up with your foot. Raise your hips and come up to a standing position.

If there is someone to help you, follow the same steps to get onto all fours. Then have the other person stand close to you, feet apart in a solid stance. Take firm hold of the person's legs in front of you, with your own hands spaced apart. Bring one knee up so your best leg is forward, and slowly crawl up the person's body to the waist. The person assisting you should not pull or push you.

Scoliosis

Scoliosis (see Chapter 3) can cause a forward flexion (tilt) of the upper body to one side. Spinal surgery is occasionally performed to correct the condition, but this is a major procedure and should be done only in exceptional circumstances. The progress of scoliosis may be slowed by an exercise program, especially if it is started early enough. Be sure to consult your physician or physiotherapist about any exercise program before you begin.

Exercises to Help Prevent Scoliosis

- Lying on your stomach, keep your right leg straight and lift it toward the ceiling. At the same time, raise your left arm. Hold this position for five seconds. Return to a relaxed position, and repeat the exercise with the left leg and right arm.
- Stand beside a wall, with the side you tilt toward closest to the wall. Place your feet about ten inches (25 cm) out from the wall. Raise the arm nearest to the wall above your head and put the other hand against the wall for balance. Now push your hip against the wall. Hold for thirty seconds and repeat five times.
- You'll need a large towel for this exercise. Sitting or standing, hold one end of the towel in your right hand. Place your right arm over your right shoulder and your left arm behind your back. Catch the other end of the towel in your left hand and pull the towel up and down five times, as if drying your back. Return to a relaxed position, reverse arms and repeat the exercise.

Leg Problems

Leg Cramps

If you tend to get leg cramps at night, be sure to sleep under loose covers to avoid pressure on your toes. A pillow at the end of the bed can be used to keep pressure off your feet. Many different devices are available at health supply stores to keep the covers off your feet.

Nightly calf-stretching exercises may be the most helpful preventive. Stand two feet from a wall. Lean forward with your hands pressed against the wall, keeping your feet flat on the floor, to give your calf a good stretch; hold and repeat. (If you're a caregiver for someone confined to bed, ask your physiotherapist to show you how to put the person's calf through a similar stretch.)

If you do have a cramp, either straighten your whole leg out and bend the foot back up toward the knee, or grab your toes and pull upward. Massage the muscles in spasm. Heat may help.

Changes in dopamine-replacement medication are often very helpful in eliminating or greatly reducing leg cramps. Quinine has been suggested as helpful, but it can have potentially serious side effects. Vitamin E and magnesium citrate or magnesium lactate have been shown to help people who do not have Parkinson's, but have not been specifically studied in those with Parkinson's.

Leg Swelling

If your legs swell, reducing your salt intake should help, since salt makes your body retain water. Also make an effort to walk more, but avoid prolonged standing.

Try to elevate your legs when you're sitting, to get gravity on your side: prop them up on a footstool, pillows or another low-seated chair. Lying down with your legs elevated for ten or twenty minutes, two or three times a day, is also most helpful.

Avoid tight stockings (knee-highs) and socks, as they restrict the flow of blood in your legs. (This does not refer to any support hose that may be recommended by your doctor.)

Note that swelling of one leg, with tenderness in the calf or pain on walking, suggests a deep vein thrombosis. This is serious because there is a risk of blood clots going to the lungs. A doctor should be consulted immediately. Deep vein thrombosis is most likely to occur in people who are more disabled, have had recent major surgery or have had a cast on.

Digestive Problems
The severity of digestive problems (especially constipation) usually relates to the duration and severity of the disability itself, rather than the treatment. Therefore, decreasing the antiparkinson medication is unlikely to be helpful. Symptoms are more likely to improve if treatment of the disability is enhanced, perhaps through the addition of further medications.

If the symptom has come on suddenly and it doesn't respond to treatment, your doctor may want to do some investigation, to rule out other possible causes.

Drooling
Frequent swallowing, instead of letting saliva pool in the mouth, is the best way to avoid drooling. Concentrate on holding your head up, deliberately closing your mouth and swallowing.
- Remind yourself to swallow by sucking a mint or chewing gum.
- Raid the kitchen spice rack; chewing a clove or simply holding a clove in the mouth for several hours can reduce drooling in some people.

Dry Mouth and Mouth Care
To avoid the discomfort of a dry mouth, try to take in more fluids, enhance saliva production and avoid dehydration. Most people manage quite well with the following suggestions:

- Drink more fluids. Sip water frequently or melt ice in your mouth.
- Use a mouth spray (either water or a commercial product).
- Suck on a mint or sour candy, or chew gum, to encourage salivation.
- Ask your pharmacist for an oral rinse, which can act as a saliva substitute.
- Take in less caffeine; it's dehydrating.
- Avoid alcohol and tobacco as they tend to dry out the mouth. (Many mouthwashes also contain large amounts of alcohol, and should be avoided for the same reason.)
- Use a humidifier in the room where you sleep.
- For dry lips, apply a lubricant such as hydrous lanolin or K-Y Jelly. Don't use a petroleum-based product, as it makes the lips dryer.
- If your tongue gets stuck to the roof of your mouth, use a straw to suck up water to lubricate your mouth; repeat as often as needed.

Dental Care

It's very important that physical disabilities not interfere with good dental care. Use proper oral hygiene techniques such as brushing teeth and flossing regularly. The caregiver should monitor dental care, and assist if necessary. Visit your dentist every six months. If tremor or poor mobility is a problem, see if you can be referred to a dentist who specializes in treating people with medical problems. Many hospitals have dental clinics.

Here are some helpful tips you can use at home.

- Lengthen or thicken the toothbrush handle with an assistive device so it's easier to hold firmly.
- If your teeth are sensitive, ask your dentist about topical fluoride gel.

- An electric toothbrush can be effective for someone with less muscle control.
- Clean dentures with a nailbrush attached to the sink with suction cups. This allows you to clean the dentures with one hand.

Difficulty Swallowing

George knew he was having problems swallowing, but he insisted that his wife, Lynn, continue serving his steak the way she always had—well done. One night at dinner, he suddenly choked on a bite of dry meat. Unable to breathe or speak, he started to panic. Lynn didn't know what to do, and she was panicking too. Fortunately, George managed to cough up the obstruction.

George reported the episode to his doctor. When he discussed it with a speech and swallowing therapist, he learned that it was easy to avoid this potentially fatal problem. As for Lynn, she took a course in CPR (cardiopulmonary resuscitation) so that she would feel confident about what to do if George ever choked again.

The best ways to avoid swallowing difficulties (dysphagia) are to eat with your chin tucked down, and to choose foods of suitable texture.

Don't rush your meals. Since eating takes longer, try four to six small meals a day instead of three larger ones. Cut your food into small pieces to make chewing easier. Always sit up to eat. To prevent food or liquid going down the wrong way, it's very important to lower your chin toward your chest and then swallow; keep your head down and swallow again. Throwing your head back to swallow may propel food or pills into your airway.

Remember to take your time; chew slowly and thoroughly. Be careful not to talk with your mouth full; using your airway while you're swallowing can lead to choking. (Home suction devices are available for people who have intermittent episodes of severe excess saliva and choking.)

Drug changes usually do little to help dysphagia, and anticholinergics may actually worsen it. However, some people only have swallowing difficulties when they are in an "off" spell; in this case, using drugs to improve motor fluctuations may significantly improve the swallowing as well. If your dysphagia is severe, it may be best to try eating only when your medications are working at their best (typically sixty to ninety minutes after you take them).

If it's not clear what's causing your dysphagia, your doctor or speech pathologist may recommend a special X-ray procedure (a *supervised barium swallow*) to pin down the specific problem.

It's possible to bypass swallowing by placing a permanent feeding tube in the stomach or upper small bowel, through a small abdominal incision. Only a few people require this, but it is a simple procedure and may greatly enhance the quality of life of someone with severe swallowing difficulties.

What if you do choke?

If you have swallowing problems, the people around you should learn the Heimlich maneuver, to clear an obstruction from a blocked airway. You may also want to learn how to do this on yourself. If you find yourself choking, make a fist and place the thumb side of that fist against your abdomen, just above the navel. Use your other hand to grasp the fist, and press inwards and upwards with quick sharp thrusts. This creates air pressure, like an artificial cough, that may blow the blockage out. Another method is to thrust your abdomen forcefully against a chairback, table, sink or hand railing to get the same effect. In either case, repeat this move until your airway is clear. Then get medical help, to be sure you are really all right.

To learn the full Heimlich maneuver, and related lifesaving techniques, sign up for a course in first aid and/or CPR. The life you save really may be your own!

The following tips may help with dysphagia:

- Take a sip of liquid after each swallow of solid food.
- To take small sips of liquid, use a straw.
- Take small sips from a full glass. This keeps your head in a better position for swallowing; tilting your head back to get the last drops makes it much harder.
- If your voice sounds wet after swallowing, swallow again.
- If you find fluids difficult to swallow, increase your fluid intake by eating jelly or sherbet, or suck on ice chips or Popsicles. You can also add thickeners to liquids to make them easier to get down; these can be obtained from most pharmacies.
- Don't mix liquids and solids in your mouth.
- Choose soft foods such as chicken, ground meat, stew, thick soup or meatloaf. Avoid hot dogs and sausages; it's too easy to choke on them.
- Put no more than half a teaspoon of food in your mouth at once.
- Foods that don't need chewing, such as yogurt and applesauce, may be placed further back on the tongue; this spares you the effort of moving the food backwards with your tongue.
- When consuming more solid foods, swallow at least twice before taking more.
- Avoid sticky foods: peanut butter, fresh white bread, dry mashed potatoes, bagels, caramel, sticky buns, thick fudge or butterscotch sauce.
- Avoid foods with small pits: olives, citrus fruits or grapes with seeds, cherries.
- Avoid foods of two or more consistencies: yogurt with fruit, soups containing lumps of solids.
- Avoid foods with stringy fibers: celery, spinach, fennel, asparagus.

- Avoid foods that don't form a mass that can be easily swallowed: most raw fruits, raisins, corn, peas, mixed vegetables, nuts, seeds, plain ground meats, dry crackers and bread, plain rice, popcorn, bran and shredded wheat cereals.
- Moisten foods with gravy, sauces, butter or cream.
- Change the consistency of foods by chopping, mincing or pureeing them with liquid to make an applesauce-like consistency.
- Use plate warmers so your food doesn't get cold. Food at room temperature may not give the sensors in your mouth much stimulation to swallow. Food should be somewhat colder or warmer than room temperature, but be careful it's not too cold or hot.
- Be sure your dentures fit properly. It's very difficult to eat if your dentures are not secure.

Constipation

Before you worry about constipation, remember that it's normal not to have a bowel movement every day. In fact, constipation is often defined as fewer than three bowel movements per week. With careful management, almost everyone with Parkinson's can manage excellent control of this bothersome component of the illness. If you develop your own individual bowel management program, and stick to it, you should be able to avoid recurring bouts of more severe constipation. A high-fiber diet, with or without laxatives, is almost always effective.

It's best to achieve this through natural means, if possible. Eat meals at regular times—colonic activity is highest in the morning and after meals, making after breakfast the best time for a bowel movement. Establish regular bowel habits—preferably thirty minutes after a meal, at the same time each day. (Recall your normal pattern, and try to return to it.) Participate in regular exercise—a ten-minute daily walk is recommended.

Increase the bulk and fiber in your diet. (But don't overdo it; too much fiber can cause bloating.) Choose:

- whole grain breads and cereals, and rice and pasta
- raw fruit, fruits with the skins, and dried fruits. If you have trouble swallowing them, try running them through a blender or food processor
- leafy vegetables: lettuce, broccoli, celery
- bran sprinkled over cereal, added to baked goods, meatloaf or casseroles.
- lentils, split peas and barley

Your body needs plenty of water to process food properly. Increase your fluid intake to four to eight glasses daily, much of it water.

- Keep drinking water near your chair.
- Don't count regular tea and coffee; the caffeine in them makes your body lose water.
- Drink fruit juices, especially prune, plum, peach and pear.
- Try senna tea.
- Remember that hot beverages, including hot water, have a laxative effect.

If these natural methods are not enough to relieve your constipation, it may be necessary to use laxatives. There are many different types available. Even if you resort to these products, continue to follow the natural steps outlined above.

- *Bulk laxatives* (such as bran, psyllium, polycarbophil and methylcellulose) increase the bulk of stool and promote easier movement of the bowels. Take one or more teaspoons twice daily in a large glass of water. *Do not use bulk laxatives if you have difficulty swallowing.* These bulking agents must be accompanied by a high liquid intake (at least eight glasses per day) or they may actually worsen constipation. Note too that abuse of laxatives can cause diarrhea.

- *Stool softeners* (such as docusate sodium) promote softer and more regular bowel movements but are only helpful for mild constipation. It takes a while before they have an effect.
- *Milk of magnesia* is something else to try, if bulk laxatives and stool softeners don't work for you.
- *Irritant laxatives* (such as mineral oil and magnesium citrate) are best avoided. Use them once per week at most; chronic use disrupts normal bowel contractions, and the bowel becomes "lazy." Long-term use of mineral oil can interfere with the body's absorption of vitamins, minerals and drugs.
- *Lactulose* helps some people. Take one to four tablespoons daily.

You may need to use a combination of the above, including both bulk laxatives and a stool softener daily. When you are

---

Fruit spread

Here's a recipe for a fruit spread that may help relieve constipation.

- ⅔ cup (150 mL) raisins
- 10 dates
- 10 dried prunes (stones removed)
- ¼ cup (60 mL) molasses
- ½ cup (125 mL) natural bran

Soak prunes in water overnight. Combine raisins, dates, prunes and prune liquid in a blender, and process well. Add molasses and bran. Transfer mixture to a casserole. Bring to a boil, then reduce heat and let simmer ten minutes. Refrigerate and serve cold. Use two tablespoons (30 mL) one to three times daily, at mealtime, on a muffin or cereal or with other food, or dissolved in hot water.

purchasing laxatives or stool softeners off the shelf, be sure to discuss the different options with the pharmacist. If constipation continues, consult your physician. Occasionally people require other drugs for constipation, or regular enemas.

Tips for Weight Loss and Poor Nutrition

Pat's wife, Louise, had Parkinson's. He was concerned about the amount of weight she was losing. He kept serving her larger and larger portions, but her weight continued to drop. When he consulted a dietitian, he learned that there were more effective ways to add calories to her diet.

Pat boosted Louise's breakfast by giving her peanut butter with her toast every day. At lunch and dinner he tempted her with small desserts—brownies and fruit tarts. Between meals and after dinner, he gave her a glass of instant-breakfast drink and a cookie. Within a month her weight began returning to a healthier level.

Weight loss can be a significant problem, particularly for people with advanced Parkinson's. Even though their caloric intake and appetite remain stable, their weight still decreases. They have to take in more calories to maintain a consistent weight.

Diet supplements are available, but they are expensive; milkshakes or "instant breakfasts" may be just as beneficial. Consider asking a dietitian to review your diet and suggest higher-calorie foods.

Eating too much carbohydrate may actually make dyskinesias worse. That's because excess carbohydrate causes the pancreas to release more insulin, which results in more of the neurotransmitter dopamine in the brain. You and your family may be able to see this effect after you have a good "sweet fix." Nonetheless, candy and other goodies should be a great enjoyment and source of calories for people with Parkinson's, and their use is encouraged. There is no evidence that it has any bad effect on the disorder.

Excess protein may make motor fluctuations worse, perhaps by causing poorer absorption of levodopa from the intestine, but more likely because it interferes with the drug's ability to enter the brain. For this reason, people with motor fluctuations are sometimes put on a low-protein diet; protein is restricted at breakfast and lunch, and most of the day's protein is taken at supper.

Before trying a low-protein diet, consult your neurologist or nurse coordinator, as well as a dietitian or nutritionist. Remember that protein adjustments will only help if you have motor fluctuations; most people just need a regular balanced diet. For that matter, the protein theory is not universally accepted. Some experts believe that once levodopa gets past the stomach and into the intestines, it's absorbed quickly, regardless of the amount of protein.

Few people stay on this diet for the long term. There are some disadvantages. If protein intake is inadequate, weight loss may result; there may be transient confusion and depression; and there will be predictable, perhaps more severe slowness following the high-protein evening meal. But if this diet is carefully managed, it may be a useful treatment option for healthy, highly motivated people with excellent nutritional status. If it is going to work, this is obvious within the first week.

If you are concerned that protein may be blocking your levodopa absorption but you don't want to try a low-protein diet, a much easier approach is to take levodopa on an empty stomach one hour before or after meals.

If you want to put on more weight, start by identifying the reasons for weight loss. If there's a swallowing problem, request a referral to a speech and swallowing pathologist to determine the cause. He or she will also give you advice to

---

Plain levodopa and vitamin B₆

If you are taking plain levodopa rather than a combination medication, excessive vitamin B₆ (pyridoxine) can be a problem. Pyridoxine can stimulate the enzyme that converts levodopa to dopamine so that, by the time the levodopa reaches the brain, it's in the dopamine form. Since dopamine can't cross the blood-brain barrier (from the bloodstream into the brain), the drug is then ineffective. Very few people are on plain levodopa, so pyridoxine is not usually an issue. If you are on plain levodopa, consult your doctor or dietitian; you should not totally eliminate this vitamin from your diet, as it plays an important role in many bodily functions.

---

make swallowing easier. If your teeth are bothering you, pay extra attention to dental care, and be sure any dentures fit properly. More frequent dental visits may be necessary. Ask yourself whether depression or anxiety is a factor; if so, talk to your doctor.

If the problem is simply that handling food is a chore, use assistive devices to make it easier, and consider having six small meals a day, so that eating takes less time and effort. Consult a dietitian about foods that are high in calories. Pay attention to preparation, so that food both looks and tastes appealing. Alternately, use your community meal service.

Remember: weight loss that begins suddenly and progresses quickly should be reported to your doctor, especially if there are other symptoms.

Bladder Problems

The first step in dealing with bladder problems is to try to identify the cause. Ask for a referral to a urologist—if possible, one with a particular interest in neurological difficulties. If a man has frequent, urgent daytime urination before he develops night-time frequency, the problem may be a flow obstruction such as prostate enlargement. An obstruction such as an enlarged prostate or a narrowed urethra may be easily fixed

---

Diuretics: the good side and the bad

While salt causes us to retain more water, certain substances make our bodies lose water, by converting it to urine. Caffeine is a very common diuretic, but many other chemicals have a diuretic effect. Diuretic pills ("water pills") are used to treat high blood pressure; when the body flushes out excess fluid, some of it comes from the blood, which reduces the pressure. Diuretics are also used for some kinds of swelling, as losing fluid reduces the swelling. But when bladder problems are causing urinary urgency and incontinence, diuretics just make things worse.

---

by a simple procedure. The trend now is away from surgery for benign prostate enlargement; more conservative treatments, including drugs, are favored (see Chapter 6).

Incontinence should also be investigated through a full urological assessment, as there is often a treatable cause. Some women have changes from childbirth resulting in urinary incontinence that can be triggered by anything that increases the pressure on the bladder—coughing or sneezing, for example. Ask a gynecologist or urologist about procedures that may alleviate the problem.

If your doctor suspects that you may also have a bladder infection, he or she may want to do a urine culture; infection is common when the bladder is not emptying completely.

Tips for Bladder Problems
- Limit fluids after dinner or if you are going out, to avoid night-time problems and embarrassing predicaments.
- Cut back on drinks with a diuretic effect, such as coffee, tea, grapefruit juice, colas and other soft drinks containing caffeine.
- Exercise your pelvic muscles to increase your retention of urine. You can improve your control by starting and then halting the flow of urine.

- If you are incontinent, you may be more comfortable using cotton underwear with liners or disposable pads. If immobility or slowness in getting to the bathroom causes night-time incontinence, keep a urinal, bedpan or commode nearby. Men can wear a condom catheter if lack of bladder control causes wetting.
- Drinking cranberry juice helps reduce unpleasant odors associated with bed-wetting or soiling of clothing.

Sexual Problems

It's not always easy to get help for sexual problems, especially if you're female. Men may be referred to urologists, who often have clinics specializing in sexual problems. A urologist may be able to help a woman, especially if she also has bladder symptoms. There should be a thorough medical examination looking for aggravating factors and any other conditions that could be contributing to the problem. Few physicians are sexual medicine consultants, so your help may come from a number of sources: your Parkinson's clinic team, family doctor, gynecologist and/or urologist. Specialty clinics often have long waits; persevere!

Dopamine-replacement medications do not tend to improve impotence directly, but they may improve mobility so that the physical act of sexual intercourse is easier. Occasionally, dopamine agonists or levodopa triggers a marked increase in sexual drive that may be accompanied by very inappropriate behavior. If this leads to significant strain on the relationship, it should be discussed with your physician; the medication can be changed.

In recent years, sildenafil (Viagra) has offered renewed hope to men with sexual difficulties. Sildenafil comes as a pill, and helps the blood vessels in the penis relax so that they can fill with enough blood to sustain an erection. Sildenafil has been shown to be safe and well tolerated, even in men with Parkinson's. The most common side effects are headache, a flushing feeling, upset stomach and visual disturbances (a blue tinge, increased sensitivity to light, and/or blurred vision). It is safe to take with most heart medications, but it must not be used in combination with nitrates (often used for chest pains or high blood pressure), or there may be a severe, potentially dangerous drop in blood pressure. Two new medications (vardenafil and tadalafil) that work in a similar way to sildenafil are expected on the market in North America in the near future. These medications take effect more rapidly and do not produce the visual disturbances associated with sildenafil.

If sildenafil is ineffective, other therapies are available: medications that can be injected into the penis or into the opening in the end of the penis, vacuum devices that draw blood into the penis, and surgically placed inflatable penile implants.

Tips for Sexual Problems
- Try to have regular sexual activity. It maintains interest and helps prevent the uncomfortable emotional feelings that can build up if sexual activity is too infrequent.
- Recognize that drugs for other problems, such as high blood pressure or anxiety, may contribute to sexual problems; consult your doctor.
- If you are depressed, treating the depression may help, but some antidepressants make sexual function worse. Be honest with your doctor about the problems you are having.
- Menopausal problems need to be addressed, as they can contribute to decreased sexual interest as well as physical difficulty with intercourse.

Above all, remember that decreased sexual function does not mean decreased love. Have an open discussion with your partner. Try to understand each other's difficulties and needs, and find ways to solve them. Chronic illness is tough on both of you, so relax, think positively, and enjoy and share each other's love in whatever ways you can.

Postural Hypotension

Some people with atypical or severe parkinsonism have a major problem with postural hypotension. Although this drop in blood pressure is usually triggered by a change in posture (such as standing up), other factors may also be involved: food, time of day, state of hydration, temperature and medication. Since blood pressure and symptoms vary over the course of the day, you need to establish the pattern of the hypotension to identify the contributing factors.

Tips for Postural Hypotension

- Review all medications with your physician, to identify any that may be contributing to the low blood pressure. Blood pressure tends to decrease slowly over the years in people with Parkinson's, so you may be able to discontinue a diuretic or other high blood pressure treatment that is no longer needed. Many cardiac drugs also lower blood pressure.
- Check for anemia (low red-blood-cell count); it is common and treatable, and can contribute to low blood pressure.
- Keep the head of your bed elevated by placing blocks of wood four to six inches (10-15 cm) thick under the legs. Alternately, use a hospital bed that tilts. Keeping your head elevated stimulates the kidneys to produce a hormone that maintains the level of salt and fluid in your bloodstream, which helps keep your blood pressure up. (Using pillows to raise your head is not as effective, as you will likely maneuver yourself into a flat position once you are asleep.)

- Avoid standing in one place too long. When standing, rock from one leg to the other, squeeze your legs together or raise your toes. All these movements tighten your leg muscles, which stops blood from pooling in your legs.
- Exercise your feet and legs before rising from a bed or chair. Cross your legs and squeeze them together to tighten your leg muscles.
- Change position slowly. After standing up, support yourself by holding onto someone or something.
- Sit down as soon as you feel faint.
- When you feel faint, raise your arms over your head for fifteen seconds. To some extent this directs blood from your arms to your brain; more important, it makes the heart pump increased blood to your brain.
- You may find elastic or support stockings useful if they cover the thigh as well as the calf. Unfortunately they are not comfortable or popular, or very effective for most people.
- Drink more fluids; dehydration lowers blood pressure.
- Drops in blood pressure are more likely after large meals, when much blood goes to the stomach to assist in digestion. It may help to eat smaller, more frequent meals.
- Increase your salt intake by adding more table salt to your food. If this is not effective, take 300 mg salt tablets (available over the counter at the pharmacy) twice a day. (Consult your physician first if you have any heart difficulties.)
- Consider having a caffeinated beverage with your meal. The caffeine constricts blood vessels, which helps keep your blood pressure up.
- If you are experiencing frequent problems with postural hypotension, avoid taking hot showers, doing excessive exercise or drinking alcohol. (Alcohol dilates the blood vessels, which lowers blood pressure.)

- Be more careful on hot days, when you sweat more and your legs swell more with fluid (edema); both of these cause the blood pressure to drop.

Shortness of Breath

Many different conditions can make you feel short of breath. Your doctor will have to investigate the problem to determine the most likely cause.

Shortness of breath is sometimes related to the use of levodopa or dopamine agonists. These drugs can cause dyskinesias; if the dyskinesias affect the diaphragm (a large muscle below the lungs that is critical to the breathing process), there may be breathing irregularities and a sensation of being short of breath. If this is the source of the problem, your doctor may try adjusting your medications.

Whatever the cause, participating in an active, ongoing exercise program will improve your breathing and cardiac (heart) function, and help you feel less short of breath. In particular, exercises to improve your chest expansion and air exchange may be beneficial. For example:

- Stand straight with your feet slightly apart, knees relaxed and arms at sides.
- Keeping your arms straight, slowly raise them out from your sides to above your head.
- At the same time, take a long, deep breath to fill your lungs with air.
- Slowly lower your straight arms in front of you, curling your back forward a little at the same time, blowing all the air out of your lungs as you do so.

Repeat this exercise three to five times daily. Stop if you feel yourself becoming lightheaded.

Skin Problems

As noted in Chapter 3, people with Parkinson's have a wide variety of skin problems, including oily facial skin, itchy eyelids (blepharitis), dry body skin and dandruff.

Tips for Facial Skin Care
- Wash the affected facial areas frequently.
- Avoid excess moisture on the face (from sweating, or not drying your face well after washing). Keep it dry and clean. It may help to limit any use of cosmetics.
- Use water-based (oil-free) moisturizing lotions and water-based makeup.
- Use a mild (drying) soap—or even baby soap—for washing your face.
- If the problem persists, see your family physician or a dermatologist. Creams containing a steroid are sometimes used for the short term, and are most helpful.

Tips for Eyelid Problems
- Apply "artificial tears" (drops that are available at drugstores without a prescription) and warm compresses three or four times daily.
- Use steroid cream if the problem is more severe.
- Use eyepatches overnight if your blinking is seriously impaired. This is to keep you from rubbing your eyes while you sleep, and perhaps scratching the corneas of your eyes.

Tips for Body Skin Care
- Limit your showers to one every second day, so your skin doesn't become too dry.
- Apply perfume-free moisturizing creams.
- Keep active with exercise and other recreation.

- Keep your weight in check. Excess skinfolds trap moisture that can lead to skin problems.
- Eat a balanced diet; it's essential for healthy skin.
- Constant pressure on one area of your skin can lead to open sores (bedsores). If you are confined to bed or a wheelchair, reposition yourself at least once every two hours. Sheepskin pads or air cushions, available at health supply stores, also help prevent bedsores.

Tips for Foot Care

It's important to maintain good foot hygiene. If foot care is difficult for you, visit a chiropodist or foot clinic. If you are not sure where to go, ask an orthopedic surgeon, or a rheumatologist with a particular interest in foot problems. It's also critical to protect feet with properly fitted shoes. Poor footwear is the most common cause of foot problems. As well:

- Wash feet once a day in warm water, but not for an extended period of time, as this would dry the feet.
- Massage feet regularly with a skin cream. Massage in an upward direction, from the toes toward the ankle. Massage should be avoided if circulation is poor, or if there is a skin infection.
- Cut toenails once a month, straight across, using clippers. This prevents ingrown toenails.
- Wear footwear that supports the feet, such as lace-up shoes with a low to medium heel. Avoid wearing slippers, as they offer little support. Don't wear restrictive footwear; the pressure may cause hard skin, bunions and corns.
- Wear socks and stockings large enough to allow movement in the toes.
- If you have cramping foot pain, consult your physician. Adjustments to your medication may relieve the problem.

Tips for Dealing with Dandruff
- Use a mild dandruff shampoo. If you prefer a stronger coal-tar shampoo, use it only twice weekly. Topical ketoconazole cream or shampoo may also be helpful; consult your pharmacist.

Visual and Eye Problems

Be sure your treatment team knows about any vision problems you are experiencing. It's vital to have the best vision you can, for both your enjoyment and your safety (good vision reduces falls and other accidents).

Start with a thorough eye exam to ensure that you have the best correction for seeing both at a distance and up close, for reading. Various aids other than eyeglasses are available to improve vision; ask your eye doctor for advice. Prisms (special corrective lenses) may help if you are having double vision. Large-print books, magnifying glasses and special reading lights make text easier to read. Devices (such as a ruler) to help you focus, stay on the line and shift to the next line can be useful. Special projection devices are also available; a book or magazine placed under the machine is projected onto a screen, making the print larger.

If you have cataracts, you may need surgery; the procedure is usually done under local anesthetic, and the improvement is often dramatic. If you have dyskinesias, there are ways to manage them during cataract surgery.

Tips for Dry Eyes
- Use a no-tears baby shampoo that won't irritate the eyes. You can also rub this shampoo into the eyelids to clean away any crusts.
- Bathe the eyes with warm water or a facecloth.
- Use "artificial tears." Pull down the lower lid and add one to two drops, three or four times daily. There are

various types of this product, so try several.
- Your doctor may prescribe an eye ointment or eyedrops.

Sweating

If excessive sweating is a problem, ask your doctor for a general review of your health and medications, to rule out causes not related to Parkinson's. Here are some practical tips that may help.
- Increase your fluid intake, especially in warm weather, to avoid dehydration.
- Keep a facecloth or towel handy.
- If your sweating is severe and you are going out, take along an extra set of clothing.
- Dress according to the weather report in winter. Otherwise, if you are feeling warm, you may underestimate how much clothing you need.
- Athletic-type clothes (track suits, T-shirts) are useful because they absorb sweat.

Speech Problems (Dysarthria)

Ruth began noticing that people frequently asked her to repeat herself. In addition, some people had difficulty understanding her on the phone. She suspected that her medication might be the reason, but it seemed to be working well otherwise, and she was not having problems with mobility.

After doing some investigation, Ruth saw a speech therapist who did the Lee Silverman type of intensive voice therapy. Within months she recognized a distinct improvement: other people no longer had to struggle to understand what she was saying, in person or over the phone.

Speech problems can be frustrating, and they can make someone with Parkinson's feel even more isolated, but fortunately there are a number of approaches you can take to

---

Speech therapy

Lee Silverman Voice Therapy (LSVT) is a form of voice treatment that teaches you to improve your speech by focusing on loudness and sensory perception. The program is intense, and requires a high degree of effort over sixteen sessions (four per week for four weeks), but it has given significant improvement that was still in effect six months later. It is done by a speech therapist, and is the only method of speech therapy to date that has been proven to work in clinical studies.

---

minimize these problems. You'll find some practical tips below. You may want to consider intensive voice treatment (see box). A referral to a speech-language pathologist (speech therapist) may also be of benefit.

General Tips for Speech
- Check that your dentures fit properly. It's very difficult to speak with loose dentures.
- If your voice is weak, try not to speak in noisy situations: in the car, on the street with traffic noises, at home with the television on, and so on. Wait until it's quieter.
- To make your speech more evenly paced, and to avoid rushes in your speech, try using a pacing device such as a "pacing board." A speech pathologist can help you with this.
- Read booklets on speech problems and suggested exercises. These are available from various Parkinson's associations.
- Speech therapy often includes exercises for the lips, tongue and jaw, to help keep your speech muscles strong. It may also help to practice facial expressions each day (smile, frown, look surprised, etc.). Look into a mirror to see how well you are doing.

Before Beginning to Speak

- Take time to organize your thoughts and plan what you are going to say.
- Practice more formal speeches. Read them aloud into a tape recorder and then play them back, listening for parts that could be improved.
- Swallow before you speak, since a lot of saliva in your mouth makes it difficult to speak clearly.
- Remember to take a breath before speaking, to keep your voice stronger.

When Speaking

- Try to keep your head upright and look at the person you are talking with. It really is easier to understand someone if you can see the mouth movements.
- Talk for yourself; don't let others do it for you.
- Express your ideas in short, concise phrases or sentences.
- Speak clearly. Every word is important. It may help to exaggerate the syllables.
- Remember to take little catch breaths as you speak; don't try to say too much on one breath. This also helps keep your voice strong.
- Use as much inflection in your voice as possible.
- Try to use as much facial expression as you can.

Other Approaches

- If your voice is extremely weak and it's very difficult for you to be heard in some situations, you may benefit from a voice amplifier. Ask your telephone company about a voice amplifier that attaches inside the speaker of your phone. A speech pathologist can provide information on the various types of voice amplifiers. Portable battery-powered models are available.

- For those whose Parkinson's is advanced, communication devices are available. These are like small typewriters; the message appears on a screen or on paper printout. Some also have voice output.
- There are operations to help weak voices by "adjusting" the tension of the vocal cords. However, the results are variable and this procedure is not appropriate for everyone. Consult a speech pathologist and/or an otolaryngologist if you want to learn more about this.

Don't shy away from telling others about the way Parkinson's has affected your speech. This may make them better listeners and allow them to help you. Educate your friends and family.

And remember—your voice may be softer now, but those around you may well be getting hard of hearing, even if they are reluctant to admit it. A hearing device might help both of you!

Other Issues

Estrogen

Parkinson's is slightly less common in women. Is this because the female hormone estrogen is a protective factor? Many different types of studies have been done to explore this possibility, but none has proven that estrogen is the reason for the difference.

Postmenopausal estrogen therapy has been suggested as a treatment that may help reduce memory problems in women with Parkinson's. Its use has been associated with a reduced risk of having Parkinson's with memory loss, and also with a reduced risk of Alzheimer's in some studies. One small study indicated that women who took estrogen after menopause were less likely to develop Parkinson's at all, but we need to do more studies before we can say for sure that estrogen reduces the risk or has a role in treating Parkinson's.

The use of estrogen by women with Parkinson's does not make their motor activity any worse, and transdermal use (wearing a "patch") may even improve it slightly. Men with prostate cancer have been treated with estrogen preparations for many years and it has not made their Parkinson's any worse. The effect of estrogen on brain cells is an area of intense research activity.

Alcohol

Alcohol has been reported, in certain studies, to have some positive effects on people with Parkinson's, including decreased tremor, improved speech and enhanced sleep. Nevertheless, alcohol is an addictive substance. For example, people who have trouble sleeping may find that alcohol promotes sleep, but it gradually loses its effect and they need to drink more and more. This leads to disruption of night-time sleep and increases their anxiety levels. Chronic, excess alcohol use can in itself lead to memory loss. As well, excess alcohol tends to cause degeneration in the cerebellum, the part of the brain that controls balance. Excess alcohol also damages the peripheral nerves, which can likewise affect balance. Because of all this, people with Parkinson's should be particularly careful to avoid drinking too much alcohol. (Also, common sense suggests that you'd better not get "tipsy" if your balance is already a bit impaired by Parkinson's.) Alcohol should never be used to treat any symptom of Parkinson's.

As noted earlier, alcohol dilates the blood vessels, so it tends to lower blood pressure. If you're having trouble with postural hypotension, you may have to stop drinking completely—at least temporarily, until your blood pressure problems are improved.

Despite all these warnings, however, a moderate amount of social drinking is a reasonable and pleasurable part of life. There is no need for most people with Parkinson's to deny themselves a drink before dinner, and a little wine with dinner. Unless your doctor has advised you to stop drinking, this is one part of your life that may remain unchanged.

Exercise and Physiotherapy

For people with Parkinson's, the goal of exercise and physiotherapy is to slow or even stop the reduction in muscle strength, joint flexibility, balance and walking ability that interferes with daily functioning. Exercise can help relieve constipation, increase energy levels, overcome sleep difficulties and slow down bone loss.

In studies, when people with moderate disability from Parkinson's followed an intensive one-month physical rehabilitation program (three sessions a week), they received measurable benefits on Parkinson's scoring scales. They improved at moving from lying to standing, making a 360-degree turn while standing, and looking over the shoulder while standing or driving. However, if they did not keep up the exercise program the benefit was lost within six months.

Exercise and your health

A twenty-two-year study of healthy middle-aged people who did not have Parkinson's showed that those who followed a moderate exercise program had a significantly reduced death rate. They had a reduction in risk factors including high blood pressure, excess body fat and high lipid (blood fat) levels, and an improvement in breathing capacity and heart function during exercise. While we focus on the special disabilities of Parkinson's, it's important to remember that people with Parkinson's also face the health risks that apply to all of us as we grow older. They too must do their best to maintain overall good health, so any reduction in their physical fitness must be vigorously opposed.

It's often preferable to attend a program outside the home, as it's not easy to persist in doing exercises on your own. This also provides an opportunity for more social interactions, and a reason to "get out of the house" and to enjoy some fresh air on the trip.

If you have Parkinson's, you should start exercising early, before you have muscle weakness, stooped posture or falls. It is much more difficult to correct these problems after they appear. You should carry out your exercise program regularly, and also do your best to continue any additional exercises or sports you enjoy. A daily walk, when weather permits, is very valuable. Physiotherapy and exercise classes are an effective and sociable form of activity. Tai chi exercise relaxes and strengthens the body, and it's gentle; even people in wheelchairs can practice it.

Try to develop a program of light to moderate exercise lasting twenty-five to thirty minutes, and carry it out daily, or at least three times per week. If possible, include some form of aerobic exercise, strength/resistance exercise, and stretching/range-of-motion exercise in your routine. Start slowly,

---

Some types of exercise

Resistance exercise involves moving specific muscles against a degree of resistance; the resistance can be provided by another muscle (pressing the palms of the hands together, for example) or by a weight or an exercise machine.

Aerobic exercise is vigorous enough that the heart and lungs must work hard to supply enough oxygen to the muscles, but not so vigorous that the body grows short of oxygen. You are in your "aerobic range" if you are slightly short of breath but still able to carry on a conversation. Aerobic exercise has to be continuous for some time (at least ten or twenty minutes) to be effective.

Passive exercise is for people who have difficulty exercising on their own. A helper gently guides the limbs through a series of movements, to keep the limbs from becoming stiff and uncomfortable.

increase at your own rate and stop if you become fatigued. It may take you several weeks to build up your stamina.

For elderly people, resistance exercises are helpful in boosting muscle strength, which contributes to better mobility and balance. Although walking is a very good form of exercise, you should also do some resistance training, including leg and arm lifts using weights and, if possible, situps to strengthen your abdominal muscles.

All the exercises described below will help develop good body fitness, but there are specific ones you can emphasize for particular problems. Develop your plan based on the advice of a physiotherapist and the suggestions outlined below. Decide what your major problems are, and give them special attention over and beyond your general program.

Shoulder and arm exercises help a frozen shoulder. Back flexibility and strength exercises can counteract stooped posture (scoliosis). Lower abdominal and pelvic exercises may help relieve constipation and urinary incontinence.

Many people with Parkinson's have bothersome hip and knee arthritis. Regular moderate exercise, either walking (aerobic) or weights and stretching (resistance), can relieve the pain and improve function. This requires a dedicated effort for thirty minutes at least three times a week.

People with more advanced Parkinson's may find some of the exercises difficult or impossible. If this applies to you, concentrate on those you can do. If you have other problems, such as heart disease, consult your physician about the level of activity best for you.

General Tips for Exercise

- Wear comfortable, loose-fitting clothing. Track suits are very popular.
- Exercise with a companion or join a group; it makes it more fun and you'll be more likely to persevere.

- Exercise to music. It will increase your enjoyment, and it may encourage you to work harder. Cassettes or CDs may be available at your Parkinson's or physiotherapy clinic, or your local library.
- Exercise at the same time every day, at the point when your medications are working at their peak.
- Start your program slowly and progress gradually over a period of weeks.
- Do all exercises slowly, in a relaxed, gentle and consistent manner.
- Never bounce when you are holding a stretch. Just feel the stretch and hold it, working up from three seconds to five or ten seconds.
- Work up to five or ten repetitions of each exercise.
- Carry a water bottle and drink regularly, to keep your fluid level up.

Home Exercise Program

While Sitting or Standing

Face:
- Raise your eyebrows and wrinkle your forehead.
- Open your mouth as wide as possible.
- Close your mouth and blow out your cheeks.
- Try to whistle.
- Wiggle your nose.
- Smile, frown and smile again.

Neck (do this slowly, in a relaxed manner):
- Tuck in your chin and place one finger on it. Draw your neck and head backward (away from the finger) as far as possible (don't tilt your head back). Hold for five seconds. Return to a relaxed position. Repeat.

- Look straight down, putting your chin on your chest. Hold for five seconds. Return to a relaxed position. Repeat.
- Turn your head to the right, looking over your right shoulder. Return your head to center, looking straight ahead. Repeat three times. Now repeat the process on the left side.
- Tilt your head to the right, bringing your right ear close to your shoulder (don't raise your shoulder). Hold for five seconds, then return your head to the upright position, looking straight ahead. Repeat three times. Now repeat the process on the left.

Shoulder:
- Put each hand on the opposite elbow to form a cradle. Lift the cradle straight up over your head, then back down.
- Rock the cradle from side to side.
- Move the cradle in large circles, first one way, then the other.
- With your arms hanging straight down, shrug your shoulders up to your ears. Return to a relaxed position.
- Raise your right arm straight up. Bend your right elbow so that your hand is hanging relaxed behind your back. Raise your left arm and grasp your right elbow with your left hand. Push your right elbow slowly and gently backwards. Return to a relaxed position. Switch arms and repeat.

Hand and wrist:
- Hold your arms straight out from your sides.
- Bending your wrists, move your hands as far as possible up and down five times.
- Bending your wrists, move your hands from side to side five times.

- Rotate your hands at your wrists, five times clockwise and five times counterclockwise. Lower your arms.
- Stretch your hands and fingers out straight. Relax.
- Squeeze your hands into fists. Relax.
- Spread your fingers apart, keeping them as straight as possible. Hold for five seconds, then bring them together. Repeat three times.
- Practice picking up coins and small objects from a table.

While Standing
Stand with your feet shoulder-width apart.

Shoulder stretch:
- Clasp your hands together behind your back. Keeping your elbows and back straight, gently raise your arms upward. Return to a relaxed position. Repeat.

Back flexibility (if your balance is unsteady, have someone standing by or hold onto a chair):
- *Corner stretch:* stand facing a corner, with one hand on each wall at shoulder height. Move your chest (not chin) toward the corner. Hold for ten to fifteen seconds. Return to a relaxed position. Repeat a few times with your hands at different heights.
- *Stooped posture exercises:* stand with your back against a wall. Press your shoulders and the small of your back against the wall. Stretch your arms to each side so that the backs of your hands are touching the wall. Slide your hands up the wall above your head, keeping arms and upper body against the wall. Return to a relaxed position. Repeat three times. Raise your right leg out in front of you as high as possible, bending it at the knee. Return to a relaxed position. Repeat with left leg. Move away

from the wall and walk with your arms clasped behind your back. Return to a relaxed position. Repeat.

- *Side stretch:* raise your arms above your head and clasp hands together. Slowly bend to the side and slightly forward until you feel a gentle stretch. Hold for three breaths. Straighten up and repeat to the other side.
- *Forward stretch:* place your hands on your hips. Keeping your back straight, gently bend forward from the waist until you feel your weight transferring to the balls of your feet (no more than 20 degrees from the vertical), hold for three seconds and then straighten up. Repeat.
- *Backward stretch:* place your hands on the small of your back, just below your waist. Slowly bend backward, as far as you can comfortably go. Hold for three seconds and then straighten up. Repeat.
- *Back rotation:* place your hands on your hips. Rotate your back to the right by looking back over your right shoulder and rotating your back to follow. Make sure your left shoulder comes forward. Hold for three seconds. Repeat on left side.

Unsteady gait exercise:

- Begin walking by lifting your right foot forward and placing the heel down first. Swing your left arm forward at the same time. Keep your head up, your shoulders back, and look straight ahead, not down. Repeat using your left foot and right arm, keeping your feet apart. Continue walking in this pattern and concentrate on swinging your arms.

While Sitting
Use a hard straight-backed chair.

Single arm stretch:

- Keeping the elbow straight, stretch your right arm over your head as high as possible. Return to a relaxed position. Repeat with left arm.

Trunk twist with arm stretch:
- Stretch your right arm out to the side with the palm facing back. Slowly twist your head, right shoulder and arm, and body to the right. Turn as far as is comfortable. Hold for five seconds. Return to a relaxed position. Repeat on your left side.

Hip stretch:
- Sit sideways on the chair, with your right arm resting comfortably on the back of the chair and your left hip on the forward edge of the seat. With your left arm, raise your left knee to your chest and then lower the leg and stretch it back behind you as far as you comfortably can. Repeat three to five times. Reverse your position and repeat with your right leg.

Hamstring stretch:
- Sit on the chair with your right foot on the floor and your left foot resting on a chair or table of equal height. Keeping your left leg straight and your arms stretched out in front, gently bend forward from the waist until you feel a comfortable stretch. Hold for three to five seconds. Return to a relaxed position. Repeat with your left foot on the floor and your right foot on the chair or table.

Leg or ankle stretches:
- Straighten out your right leg and hold for five seconds. Return to a relaxed position. Repeat three times. Repeat with left leg.

- Starting with your feet flat on the floor, raise your bent right knee up as far as possible and then lower your foot to the floor. Repeat three times. Relax and repeat with your left knee.
- Extend and flex your right ankle, as in a flutter-kick. Repeat three times. Repeat with left ankle.
- Make large circles with your right foot. Repeat with left foot.

While Lying on Your Back

Lie on a firm, comfortable surface such as a carpeted floor or a firm bed. Use a small cushion to support your head and neck. During the exercises, try to keep the small of your back pressed against the bed or floor. Discontinue the exercises if they cause or aggravate back pain.

Pelvic tilt:
- Bend your knees and place your feet flat on the bed or floor. Push the small of your back down to the surface by tightening your lower abdomen. Hold for three to five seconds. Relax and repeat.
- Raise your hips off the surface. Hold for three to five seconds. Relax and repeat.

Upper abdominals:
- Bend your knees and place your feet flat on the bed or floor. Flatten your back against the surface as in the pelvic tilt. Reach your arms over your knees and pull your shoulder blades up from the bed or floor. Hold for three to five seconds. Return to a relaxed position. Repeat.

Oblique abdominals:
- Lie as in the pelvic tilt. Reach both arms slowly to the right, to the outside of your knees, raising your head and

shoulder blades off the bed or floor. Hold for three to five seconds. Return to a relaxed position. Repeat to the left of your knees.

Front thigh stretch:

- Bend your knees. Keeping the small of your back pressed against the bed or floor, grasp your right knee with both hands and bring it up to your chest. Stretch your left leg out and press it against the bed or floor. Hold for three to five seconds. Return to a relaxed position. Repeat with left knee and right leg.

Back thigh stretch:

- Stretch your arms above your head. Raise your right knee. Straighten out your right leg and stretch your heel to the ceiling. Point your toes toward the ceiling. Return to a relaxed position. Repeat with the left knee.

Back stretch and relaxation:

- Lie with your legs out straight and your arms at your sides, palms facing up. Flatten your back to the bed or floor. Try to relax, letting the muscles stretch to allow your arms and legs to straighten out. Breathe deeply and relax for five to fifteen minutes.

While Lying on Your Side

For thighs, hips and waist:

- Lie on your right side with your right leg bent. Rest your head comfortably on your extended right arm. Place your left hand on the bed or floor at waist level to keep your balance. Keeping your left leg straight and your toes pointed forward, slowly raise and lower the leg as far as possible. Repeat three to five times. Turn over onto your left side and repeat.

Hip exercises:
- Lying on your right side with your right leg slightly bent, raise your left leg about 30 degrees and move it forward in front of you, keeping it straight. Hold for five seconds. Return to a relaxed position. Repeat three to five times.
- Still lying on your right side, cross your left leg over your right to rest on the bed or floor in front of you. Keeping your right leg comfortably straight, raise it toward the ceiling, keeping your toes pointed forward. Hold for five seconds and relax slowly. Repeat three to five times.
- Turn onto your left side and repeat these two exercises.

While Lying on Your Stomach
Place a small pillow under your abdomen for comfort.

Arm lifts for stooped posture:
- Stretch your arms out past your head on the bed or floor. Raise your right arm as high as possible and turn your head to look at it. Lower your arm. Do the same with your left arm. Repeat three to five times.

Leg strengthening exercise:
- Resting your head comfortably on your folded arms, raise your right leg about six inches above the bed or floor, keeping the knee as straight as possible. Lower the leg slowly. Repeat with left leg. Repeat exercise three to five times.

Knee exercise:
- Bend your right knee as far as possible, bringing your right foot toward your buttock and keeping your thighs against the bed or floor. Hold for three to five seconds and straighten out slowly. Repeat three to five times. Repeat the exercise with left knee.

Passive Exercises

When someone has long periods of immobility, passive exercises can help to prevent stiff muscles and joints and promote comfort. The helper simply lifts and moves the arms, legs and neck in gentle movements that imitate normal actions. These can be taught by a physiotherapist.

- While the person is sitting, raise both his or her arms above the head and lower them.
- Straighten the person's legs, while he or she is still sitting.
- Turn the person's head gently from side to side.
- Lower the person's head gently down toward the chest and raise it back up.

Do not attempt the following unless you are confident that you yourself will not fall, and the person you are helping has no history of falling.

- Stand in front of the sitting person. Brace your feet firmly, with your toes touching the other person's, to avoid slipping. Grasping his or her hands, raise the person to a standing position. Raise the arms above the head. Lower the person back down.

Community Services

Most people with Parkinson's, and their families, need outside help at one time or another in coping with the difficulties and complexities of this long-term disability. When problems arise, feel free to discuss them with your doctor or nurse, so that you can be referred to the appropriate community services. These services allow people to live at home longer, and help improve their quality of life. They also provide much-needed relief to caregivers. Many of these services are covered under private medical insurance or government health plans. The types of services and number of hours of help you can receive vary, depending on your level of disability and the availability of the services locally. The following are examples of services that may be available in your community.

Home Care

This program is for people who need professional health care at home. Your doctor can refer you to the program, and then a coordinator will probably interview you in your home and refer you to whatever specific services are appropriate. Services typically include nursing, physiotherapy, occupational therapy, speech therapy, social work, nutritional counseling and homemaking.

Meal Services

If you are unable to prepare your own meals, you may be able to have ready-to-reheat meals delivered to your door. The service typically arrives in the morning and supplies three meals for the day, five days a week.

Visiting Nurses

This service is often provided through your local home-care agency. Registered nurses come to your home, under a physician's orders, to give general nursing care, supervise medication, check blood pressure, change dressings and carry out other medical duties.

Professional Homemaking Services

These homemakers assist people who wish to continue living on their own. They provide help with shopping, do some housekeeping, and assist with meal preparation and personal care.

Day Hospital Programs

These programs provide care and treatment (physiotherapy, speech therapy, craft programs, etc.) for disabled people in a hospital setting during the day, a few days per week, depending on need. This allows the person to maintain daily activities and receive rehabilitation and support services. It also gives the caregiver some assistance and free time.

Respite Care Programs
Respite care allows the disabled person and the caregiver to have a vacation from each other. For example, the disabled person may spend one month in a hospital or lodge and then two months at home. The length of stay varies. You may even be able to plan a stay at the same time each year.

Permanent Placement
Permanent placement homes can be found in the directory of resources in your community (see below). They are usually nursing homes, homes for the aged and chronic care hospitals. Waiting lists are long, so it's important to anticipate the need and act upon it before the situation becomes critical. Your home-care program may be able to help you find a suitable facility.

Transportation Services
Special transportation services are often available for those who can't drive or take a regular bus because of a disability. Ask your local transportation service about this. You may also be able to get a "handicapped" sign or sticker for the family car. These generally allow you to park in some (not all) areas that are otherwise "no parking," and in "handicapped only" zones. Ask your local motor vehicle registration unit how you can apply for one. An application for either disabled transport or a handicapped sticker will have to be signed by your doctor.

Parkinson's Associations
These associations offer information, education and support to people with Parkinson's, and their family and friends as

well. They can provide information on such topics as income tax deductions, drug benefit plans, assistive devices, social services and other benefits. They also raise money for research and patient care. All in all, they are a very important component of the total care program. If someone in your family has Parkinson's, the family should belong to the local organization.

Directory of Resources for Senior Citizens

For many communities, there is a directory of the services that may be helpful to senior citizens. It's similar to a phone book, although it provides more detail about each service. The directory is often available through the local senior citizens' council, but seniors are not the only ones who can benefit from this informative book.

Managing Hospital Stays

When it's necessary for someone with Parkinson's to be admitted to hospital—for surgery or some other reason—the routines of daily living, and particularly the medication schedule, are overthrown by the hospital timetable and other disruptions. With forethought and careful attention to detail, most problems can be avoided, sparing everyone a lot of distress.

Medication

The most common problem, when a person with Parkinson's is admitted to the hospital, is often the medication schedule. Medications may need to be given very frequently, with varying doses and at quite specific times. In addition, some people find that their medications work better if taken thirty minutes prior to a meal, or find that they tolerate them better when they take them after a meal. For most medications that nurses give, there are fairly rough timelines (eight a.m., noon, five p.m., bedtime) and therefore nurses don't always realize that being a half-hour too early or too late can mean a marked difference to someone with Parkinson's.

To assist the hospital staff, it's important that you have a current list of your medications and dosages, and an easy-to-follow medication schedule. Just bringing in the pill bottles may not be enough, especially if you forget to tell staff that the timing instructions have changed from what's on the bottle. As well, many Parkinson's medications come in different-sized tablets, and some also come in a slow-release form; an inadvertent substitution can cause problems.

It's important that all this be discussed in detail at the time of admission, so that there are no misunderstandings and so that you and the staff don't become frustrated with each other. Although most institutions prefer to administer all medications, when a patient has a complex schedule it is often possible for the patient or caregiver to manage the medications, to ensure that everything is done on time.

Confusion

People with Parkinson's are more susceptible to confusion than other people being admitted to the hospital. Anyone undergoing surgery can develop postoperative confusion and delirium, but those with Parkinson's are at higher risk. Risk factors for confusion include:

- preexisting memory loss or confusion
- older age
- dopamine-replacement medications

For most patients with Parkinson's this postoperative confusion is limited, lasting only a day or two. As a general anesthetic creates a higher risk of confusion, a local anesthetic should be used if at all possible. Postoperative pain needs to

Strategies for helping a patient with preexisting memory difficulties
- Reorient the person, gently but frequently.
- Try to ensure that he or she sleeps well.
- For anyone with visual or hearing impairment, make sure eyeglasses, magnifiers and hearing aids are brought to the hospital.
- Prevent dehydration by ensuring that adequate liquids are easily accessible.

be treated adequately, but all pain medications can increase confusion so they should be used cautiously.

If confusion is a significant problem, it may be necessary to temporarily lower the dosage of Parkinson's medication. Many of the drugs given to control delirium (neuroleptics) block dopamine in the brain. In the hospital, older "typical" dopamine-blocking drugs (for example, haloperidol) are frequently used, but they can dramatically worsen the mobility of someone with Parkinson's. If medications are needed to control delirium, only the newer "atypical" neuroleptics should be used. Quetiapine and clozapine appear to be the best tolerated.

Deep Vein Thrombosis
Deep vein thrombosis (blood clots in the veins) can happen to anyone who has prolonged immobility. It typically occurs in the legs, and causes swelling of the affected leg. This can be very uncomfortable, but a greater concern is that part of the clot may break free and travel to the lungs, causing shortness of breath or even death. As people with Parkinson's already have problems with their mobility, they are at greater-than-average risk when admitted to hospital. Provided that the hospital staff recognize this, the problem can normally be prevented easily with proper care. It's important to maintain the person's mobility as much as possible, through proper med-

ication management. Aggressive physiotherapy is also essential. If prolonged immobility cannot be avoided, medications can be given to thin the blood and discourage clots.

Pneumonia

Pneumonia (infection of the lungs) is another common problem for anyone admitted to hospital, but people with Parkinson's are at increased risk, for two main reasons. They can have more difficulty generating a deep cough to avoid accumulating fluid in the lungs. In addition, they may have trouble swallowing, in which case there is a danger of food or drink accidentally entering the airway and reaching the lungs. Extra instructions from the nurses, respiratory therapist and speech/swallowing therapist can be very helpful (see "Difficulty Swallowing," earlier in this chapter).

Slow Recovery

Try to accept the fact that recovery time is generally longer for people with Parkinson's. An extended recuperation time should be expected and planned for, so that you don't become overly concerned or frustrated about the delay. You will need to work harder than the average patient who has had a similar surgery or medical problem to recover your previous level of functioning.

Remember, just because you have Parkinson's doesn't mean you won't have anything else. If you remain as physically active as you can, it will help you recover from whatever other health problems may come along.

FIVE

Social Aspects of Parkinson's

For much of human history, people with physical handicaps were cut off from many aspects of life. Depending on the nature of the handicap, they might be unable to work, to travel, even to leave home. Not any more! As our society becomes more inclusive, and as technology becomes more sophisticated, people with serious disabilities are enjoying activities and freedoms that would have been impossible even twenty-five years ago.

Pregnancy

Because so many drugs are used to treat Parkinson's, a pregnancy in a woman with the disorder raises difficult questions about what effects her medications may have upon her child. The whole question of pregnancy should be discussed in detail by both prospective parents, and with the physician, preferably before the woman becomes pregnant. The discussion should include the stage of her disease, the exact diagnosis and the prognosis (anticipated progression of the disease). Although the progression of Parkinson's in younger people varies widely, overall it tends to be slower than when the disease begins at an older age.

Fewer than fifty pregnancies have been reported in Parkinson's patients. Despite this limited base of knowledge, some helpful guidelines and findings are available.

Animal studies have shown that levodopa can cause fetal abnormalities including low birth weight and liver, heart and bone problems. All dopamine agonists in high doses have been shown to lower pregnancy rates. Among them, pergolide, bromocriptine and pramipexole seem safe, but high doses of ropinirole may cause reduced survival rates and abnormalities of the fingers and toes in lab animals. The MAOI selegiline is associated with an increase of miscarriages and still births, and amantadine clearly causes malformations in animals.

Human experience shows that Parkinson's may worsen during pregnancy and may not improve after delivery. Therefore, if the mother is already on antiparkinson medication, stopping it may not be a good option. Levodopa use during human pregnancy has not been associated with any major maternal problems, but one case of osteomalacia (bone softening) in an infant has been reported. Bromocriptine has been widely used to facilitate pregnancy in women with prolactin disorders who did not have Parkinson's—prolactin is a hormone involved in breastfeeding, among other things, and its production is affected by dopamine—and was used in at least one woman who did have the disease, and all was well. There is similar but more limited experience with pergolide in women without Parkinson's. So far there are no reports of pramipexole being used in pregnant women, and the manufacturer recommends caution; however, animal studies have shown no problems. But major birth defects have been reported in humans following the use of amantadine, and there are no reports on selegiline; neither of these two drugs should be used by a woman who is pregnant.

> ## Levodopa and breastfeeding
> Levodopa is excreted in breast milk. The concentration of the drug is small, and will be as low as possible if feedings (or breast-pump use) can be coordinated with the drug schedule. The levels of both regular and slow-release levodopa preparations peak about three hours after the drug is taken, and return to minimum about three hours after the peak—so levels may be lowest just before the medication is taken, or at least six hours after.

It's quite feasible for a woman to breastfeed while on antiparkinson therapy. Dopamine agonists interfere with lactation, so they probably should not be used, but amantadine shows up in breast milk in very low amounts, and no infant problems have been reported. We don't know whether selegiline is excreted in breast milk. Levodopa does appear in breast milk, but the dose the infant receives is very small and no problems have been reported.

Our experience with Parkinson's in human pregnancy is limited. However, by combining our knowledge of both animals and humans, we can come up with the following general guidelines.

- Parkinson's may worsen during pregnancy.
- You should not suddenly stop taking any drug.
- During pregnancy, levodopa is probably safe, but experience with animals suggests caution; it seems best to avoid the drug if possible.
- During pregnancy, amantadine and selegiline should not be used.
- Dopamine agonists seem safe, judging from extensive use among women without Parkinson's. We have no human experience with pramipexole or ropinirole, but ropinirole should not be used because of abnormalities in the animal studies.
- Levodopa is safe for the nursing infant. Amantadine is probably safe for the nursing mother and infant. Dopamine

agonists may reduce lactation but some mothers have nursed while on them.

Even in the face of Parkinson's, both parents can share the joys of child-rearing, but they will need big doses of humor, mutual support and understanding. They will also need to be honest with the child, as far as the child's age permits. The child should learn to be helpful and independent as early as is possible without overburdening either the child or any older siblings. Show hope and optimism, not sadness and self-pity. With a positive family approach, your children will grow up well equipped to handle other crises in life. As one Parkinson's mother reports, you will be rewarded with comments like "Mom doesn't smile as much as before [because of reduced facial expression], but she always smiles in her heart."

Employment

Many people develop Parkinson's when they are still young and employed. With some adjustments, and with the support of family and co-workers, they can continue working. This not only helps them financially, but also enhances their feelings of independence and self-worth. With good medication management and support, many people enjoy years of productive, rewarding work after their diagnosis.

Tips about Employment

- Inform your employer and co-workers that you have Parkinson's. This will prevent any obvious symptoms from being misinterpreted. For example, tremor might be mistaken for excessive nervousness during presentations.
- Discuss with your physician the timing of your medication, so that the more stressful hours of work are covered.

- Request a referral to an occupational therapist who can assist you with techniques and equipment to make tasks easier.
- To help cope with writing difficulties, make use of computers, typewriters, dictating units, and pen or pencil grips.
- Ask your employer about the possibility of reduced or flexible hours, or a transfer to less demanding work.
- If you become unable to work, be very aware of your disability coverage and pension before any final decisions are made. Discuss this with both the human resources people in your company, and someone outside, like your insurance broker or financial planner.
- Never accept Parkinson's-related termination or layoff if it is not to your advantage. Consult a lawyer or a human rights organization if necessary.

Driving

The benefits of comfort, convenience and freedom that come from being able to drive your own vehicle are well recognized. However, these mean little when they are measured against our legal and moral obligation to avoid hurting other people. It has been shown that people with moderately severe Parkinson's are involved in about ten times more traffic accidents than people of the same age in the general population.

Studies show that people whose Parkinson's causes this level of disability drive more slowly, don't maintain good lane position, and make more mistakes when their attention is divided. Because of their slower reactions, it may take them one-third longer to react to a situation and bring the car to a safe stop. As a result of all this, they tend to have more rear-end collisions and sideswiping accidents.

In addition to the effects of the Parkinson's itself, people with this disorder may be taking many drugs that also affect their ability to drive safely.

Recognizing declining driving skills

Much as we may treasure the independence of driving, it's vital to give up the wheel before Parkinson's causes an accident, perhaps a serious one. Signs of poor driving include:

- driving too slowly for the conditions
- making turns that are too wide or too sharp
- not heeding traffic signs or signals
- making an excessive number of minor errors

Anyone with Parkinson's who is involved in a motor accident should be very thoroughly reviewed with regard to driving skills.

It's no secret that most of us overestimate our own driving capability. For that reason, it's important to be realistic about the risks involved, and to listen to the concerns of others. If you are more uneasy driving than you used to be—if your family have doubts about your driving—if you have had an accident or a near-miss—it's time to consult your doctor about whether you are still safe on the road. Most regions require physicians to report individuals with any medical problems that may impair their ability to drive safely.

If you feel you are still able to drive, take measures to reduce your risk. Drive only in daylight, in good weather. Try to stay on side streets and back roads, where speeds are slower and traffic is lighter. Consider enrolling in a defensive driving course, which will remind you about the fine points of driving and collision avoidance. Avoid distractions: stay off the cellphone, turn off the radio and keep conversation to a minimum.

If you are wondering whether you should continue to drive, the following points may help you decide.

- Having Parkinson's does not necessarily mean you are unsafe to drive.
- If you have more severe disability (Hoehn and Yahr stage III) you probably should not be driving; if you do still drive, take the precautions listed above.

- If your driving makes you or your family feel unsafe, you should not be driving.
- Remember that motor fluctuations and medication side effects decrease your coordination and increase your risk. Be especially cautious when you are starting a new medication or moving to a higher dose.
- Using a taxi may feel expensive at the time, but car expenses (and parking fees) add up. If you take the time to calculate the total cost of running your car, you may find that taxis are a very practical alternative.
- If you (or others) are doubtful about your driving ability, take a repeat driving test or a driving skill assessment. Most driving schools will do road tests and give you an independent assessment of your skills. Some rehabilitation centers offer very detailed off-road assessments that include memory testing and reaction times, in addition to an on-road test. Let an expert make the decision.

If you must stop driving, try to accept the decision with good grace, difficult as that may be. Your safety and the safety of others—not to mention your conscience and peace of mind—are far more important than the privilege of driving.

Travel

Even people with very significant disabilities may travel quite well. Indeed, when people with Parkinson's travel south in the winter, they usually feel better in the warmer climate. There's no need to miss out on this stress-relieving activity because of your disabilities.

As the population ages, and more and more people are traveling with disabilities, the travel and service industries are adapting. More locations such as hotels and museums are wheelchair accessible, and so are some taxis. There are books, organizations and Internet websites devoted to supplying information for travelers with disabilities. See Further Resources, at the end of this book, for more information.

Take Your Medical History with You

Be sure to take along a letter stating your medical problems. Find the name and address of a neurologist or general practitioner at your destination; your doctor or a friend already living in the area can help with this. Once you arrive, check the location of the hospital and other medical facilities, in case of emergency. Also check whether there's an emergency phone number (such as 911).

Take time to review the conditions of your health insurance. You may need extra travel health insurance to cover cash payments out of the country. Be sure to carry photocopies of any health insurance documents you may need.

Think Ahead about Medications

Bring enough medication for the holiday; you may have difficulty getting your prescriptions filled when you are out of your own state, province or country. And be sure to carry your medication with you. Do not put it in your checked luggage, which may be stolen or misrouted. Bring extra medication, and consider splitting it between two carry-on bags, in case of loss or theft. You may also need a copy of your prescriptions, or a letter documenting your medications from your doctor, so you don't have trouble taking your drugs across the border. You won't normally need this within North America, but you could have problems if you are traveling abroad. Also make sure that you remember or take with you the generic names of all your drugs, as the brand names may be different in another country.

Tips for the Trip

- Prebook your airline (or train) seat and explain your disabilities for extra service. On an airplane a bulkhead seat may be more private but, depending on the plane, may also give you less leg room. You may want a seat closer to the washroom if you have bladder difficulties.

- Wheelchairs are available, and airline personnel are very helpful. They may also know the shortcuts around the airport.

- Travel by car and bus can also be practical and enjoyable, if the trip is carefully planned to have shorter drives and more stopovers than usual.

- If you are flying overnight, you may want to continue your levodopa doses every three to four hours, as you do in the daytime.

- Leg and foot swelling (edema) is common during long flights. Wear loose-fitting shoes (preferably with laces). Move your legs frequently when sitting; flex and extend your feet. Get up and move about if possible. Try to elevate your legs as much as possible. Drink only small amounts of alcohol as this can lead to dehydration. All of these points will help you avoid deep vein thrombosis (blood clots) in the legs, which is a risk with prolonged immobility.

SIX

Treating Parkinson's: Drugs and Surgery

The Issues of Drug Therapy

We have an increasing number of medications to treat the symptoms of Parkinson's, but unfortunately none of those currently available clearly slows the progression of the disease. It was originally claimed that selegiline did so, but most of the evidence now indicates that it really only seems to reduce the symptoms.

How Early Should Symptoms Be Treated?

In the early stage of Parkinson's, when symptoms are noticeable but not troublesome, symptomatic treatment is not necessary—and therefore, since all drugs have the potential to induce side effects, treatment is not usually recommended. As a general rule, it is appropriate to start treatment when the person begins to experience functional difficulties that result in

- a reduced quality of life
- impaired performance of activities of daily living
- inability to work effectively

This decision about when to begin drug therapy varies with the person; we all have different views of how much functional impairment it takes to reduce our quality of life. However, it has been shown that, when effective treatment of symptoms is delayed beyond the point where there is significant disability, the person is likely to survive for a shorter time.

What Drugs Should Be Used?

There is no simple answer to this question. Therapy may begin with a less potent (and less effective) agent, such as selegiline, amantadine or one of the anticholinergics. When these no longer do enough to relieve the symptoms, levodopa is still considered the most effective therapy. But because so many different drugs are available, treatment decisions are complex, and therapy must be tailored to each patient individually. For example, because younger people are more likely to have motor complications, they may benefit from delaying the use of levodopa; when more potent therapy is needed, they may be better off with early treatment with a dopamine agonist.

How Is the Dosage Decided?

To keep side effects to a minimum, it's important to start these drugs slowly, and work up gradually to the dose that is needed. It's generally wise for older people to start with even smaller doses, make slower increases and be especially watchful for adverse side effects. If one drug does not seem to be helping at all, that therapy should be ended before another is started. Drugs interact with each other; the more drugs you are taking, the more side effects are likely. Most people with moderate

---

Drugs are not a "do-it-yourself" project!

It's helpful to understand what drugs you are taking and why, and what side effects may result. You should feel free to ask questions about your drugs, and even suggest changes to your family doctor or neurologist. But you should not change your drug regimen on your own. Any changes *must* be decided in consultation with your doctors.

---

parkinsonian disability require several drugs to control their symptoms, but *unnecessary* combinations should be avoided.

In the sections that follow, drugs are identified by their generic names. For company brand names, please see the table at the end of Chapter 7.

Levodopa

Levodopa (often called L-dopa) is converted to dopamine in the brain. (Dopamine is the chemical that is deficient in the brains of people with Parkinson's. Dopamine itself cannot be used as therapy, because it cannot easily cross into the brain; levodopa can.) Levodopa helps reduce rigidity and tremor, and is most effective in combating bradykinesia (slowness of movement). It's the mainstay of treatment for Parkinson's, and the best drug available. Almost anyone can take levodopa, and almost everyone with Parkinson's will eventually be treated with it.

The Levodopa Debate

With time, some people with Parkinson's develop symptoms that respond poorly to levodopa therapy, such as speech and cognitive difficulties, certain problems with walking, and postural instability. In addition, a variety of motor complications (see "Major Side Effects of Levodopa," below) occur *in association with* using levodopa. We don't really understand what causes these complications, but they are one reason for the longstanding debate over whether levodopa treatment should be delayed. The other reason is the concern that levodopa may damage the brain's dopamine cells (see box).

When people with a normal dopamine system (e.g., those with essential tremor) are treated with levodopa, they do not develop these levodopa-related motor complications, even after prolonged exposure. Parkinson's patients did not have these types of motor fluctuations prior to the discovery of levodopa, but they were recognized soon after the drug was introduced. The dose of levodopa clearly plays a role, since the abnormal movements improve or resolve when the dose is lowered.

The duration of treatment also contributes to these motor problems; in one study, complications increased from 20 percent in the first five years to 70 percent after fifteen years of treatment. The "pulsatile stimulation" of dopamine receptors by levodopa is also felt to play a role. Levodopa is given

Levodopa and toxicity

Some reports have been published that levodopa may be toxic to dopamine cells. The evidence for this is derived mainly from experiments in which dopamine cells were grown in isolation and levodopa was placed with them; dopamine cells exposed to high concentrations of levodopa died faster than cells not exposed. However, if the experiments are repeated with the addition of the normal supporting cells found in the brain, this toxic effect is not seen, and the predominant effect may in fact be protective. Studies in healthy animals have consistently failed to demonstrate that levodopa is toxic, and indeed it has been shown to prolong the lifespan of some mice.

No studies in humans have shown that long-term administration of levodopa damages dopamine cells. Autopsies of non-parkinsonian patients exposed to levodopa for many years have revealed no damage to their dopamine cells. Human studies have clearly shown that levodopa improves the life expectancy of people with Parkinson's, but this may be a result of its marked beneficial effect on disability, rather than a true slowing of the disease's progression.

intermittently and its effect within the brain is short-lived, so its action on the dopamine receptors is temporary. There is a theory that this pulsatile or on-off stimulation may actually change the cells receiving the dopamine signal, so that they become excessively activated by each signal. One reason why dopamine agonists are less likely to cause dyskinesias may be the fact that they act over a longer period of time.

The person's age at the onset of the disease also affects the occurrence of these problems. People with young-onset Parkinson's (under the age of forty) have a greater risk of developing dyskinesias and motor fluctuations, and this has encouraged many neurologists to delay the introduction of levodopa as long as possible for people in this group.

Overall, it remains unknown whether the motor complications seen with long-term levodopa therapy are exclusively the result of that therapy, or are more related to the progression of the disease. We can hope that studies currently underway will resolve this issue.

How Levodopa Is Taken

Levodopa is commonly used in combination with either carbidopa or benserazide, because these drugs help stop the levodopa from changing to dopamine before it reaches the brain. These combination preparations are more effective than plain levodopa, and allow us to use about 80 percent less levodopa—which helps reduce side effects of nausea, low blood pressure (postural hypotension) and heart problems.

Controlled-release levodopa/carbidopa is very helpful for the fluctuating symptoms of Parkinson's; it dissolves slowly in the stomach, so its effect lasts longer. It can give longer periods of mobility ("on" time) and a more predictable day. This combination is very useful for end-of-dose failure (the "wearing off" effect—see below), as the total number of doses per day can often be reduced.

Tips for taking levodopa

- Take the medication after a light snack or meal, to reduce side effects.
- If fluctuations are a problem, it may help to avoid taking levodopa after a high-protein meal. Amino acids (which make up proteins) may slow the absorption of levodopa, and may block its transport into the brain.
- Chew regular levodopa/carbidopa tablets if you want quicker onset of action, unless nausea is a problem. Do not crush or chew controlled-release tablets.
- Chronic mild nausea may improve if you change to a levodopa compound with more carbidopa or benserazide.
- It is quite reasonable to adjust the timing (but not the quantity) of your doses of plain levodopa to suit your own fluctuations and life pattern. Tell your doctor or clinic nurse of any changes on each visit.
- A mid-evening dose of levodopa may help when you are spending the evening out.
- A very early morning dose of levodopa may help morning slowness or leg and foot cramps.

The main problem with controlled-release levodopa/carbidopa has been the slower onset of action compared to regular levodopa/carbidopa. The overall daily dose of levodopa has to be increased by about 30 percent because the levodopa is not completely absorbed. Other methods are now being studied to improve the effectiveness of levodopa in people whose response to the drug fluctuates severely; these include injectable levodopa, and rapidly dissolving oral forms.

Levodopa should be started slowly, taken after food, and gradually increased to a low therapeutic dose; that level should be maintained until the benefits can be assessed. Less fatigue, improved general well-being, faster movements and better walking are usually the first benefits. Tremor improves less.

Minor Side Effects of Levodopa
Minor side effects include initial mild nausea, which usually clears quickly, anorexia (loss of appetite for food), and dis-

---

Levodopa and melanoma

When levodopa was first being used, there was some concern that it could trigger the appearance or recurrence of melanoma (serious skin cancer). Long-term experience has shown that this is not true. Levodopa does not increase the risk of melanoma, even in people who have previously had the problem. It may even reduce the likelihood of the disease. Studies are underway to try to determine whether people with Parkinson's have a higher risk of skin cancers in general. The literature published so far on the subject is controversial.

---

turbed sleep and/or upsetting dreams. More severe stomach upset may be reduced by taking small doses after food; if this does not help, the drug domperidone should be used. Most of the levodopa does not actually reach the brain, but is converted to dopamine in other parts of the body. This extra dopamine can lead to nausea and lower blood pressure. Domperidone blocks these side effects outside the brain but it can't cross into the brain, so it has no effect on the dopamine levels there. Changing from levodopa/carbidopa to levodopa/benserazide (or vice versa) occasionally improves severe stomach upset, or the rare occurrence of diarrhea, caused by starting levodopa.

Levodopa rarely causes confusion initially; if it does, the drug should be reduced or temporarily stopped and all drugs should be reviewed.

Major Side Effects of Levodopa

Daily Mobility Fluctuations
Initially, the improvement with levodopa seems even and stable over the course of the day. After years of treatment, however, people begin to notice a return of their parkinsonism three to five hours after their last dose. This fluctuation is more common and severe in younger patients. Levodopa absorption varies considerably throughout the day, and it seems that the absorption becomes less consistent in the afternoon and

evening, which can lead to this worsening of symptoms. In addition, over the long term there are changes in the way the brain stores and handles dopamine, because of the loss of dopamine nerve terminals; handling of levodopa in the rest of the body is also altered. There are several types of mobility fluctuations.

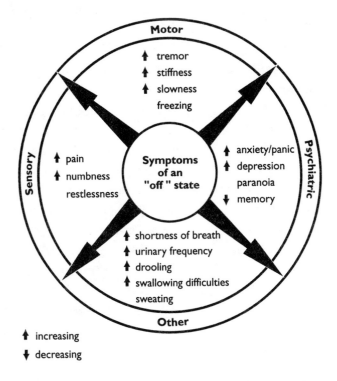

End-of-dose failure ("wearing off" effect): parkinsonian symptoms return before the next dose of levodopa is due. This may not occur after each dose; it is more common later in the day, and may be delayed for five to six hours in the first few years of treatment. It is most likely related to the state of the dopamine-producing cells in the brain when the treatment is started. With a greater loss of cells and a lower level of dopamine, end-of-dose failure may be more prominent. Even the nature of this loss of effect may vary from person to person. Some people have a subtle increase in slowness or tremor; others become completely unable to walk.

Relief of these disabilities usually comes only with the next dose of levodopa, and then not until that dose is absorbed from the stomach and reaches the brain (after thirty to sixty minutes). This delay is sometimes misinterpreted; people may feel that their drugs sometimes make them briefly worse.

"On-off" phenomenon: the beneficial effects of levodopa therapy may rapidly, unpredictably appear and disappear, as the person fluctuates from mobility to sudden immobility. The mobile or "on" phase is the condition of responding optimally to the medications. During such periods, someone can move about and perform activities of daily living with relative ease. This phase is commonly accompanied (or disturbed) by dyskinesias. The "off" phase is the period of time when someone is having more difficulty with movement.

The "on-off" phenomenon is the most severe type of fluctuation, and typically occurs much later in the course of the disease. This fluctuation is unpredictable and is not clearly related to the timing of levodopa doses.

Freezing: these sudden, brief (seconds-long) periods of immobility are felt to be more part of the illness than a levodopa complication. They may occur during levodopa "wearing-off spells," in which case they respond to increased medication. They may also occur during "on times," in which case they respond poorly to drug changes, and may actually be worsened by increasing doses of levodopa.

No "on" response: fluctuating patients whose disease is advanced occasionally fail to respond to a dose of levodopa. This condition of not having an "on" response is usually due to inadequate absorption of levodopa, and may be caused by an inadequate dose, by slow passage of the drug through the

> ## Motor fluctuations and menstruation
> In some women, motor fluctuations may be up to 50 percent worse for a few days before and during menstrual periods. This worsening has been improved remarkably with acetazolamide, taken just before and during menstruation.

gastrointestinal tract due to the effects of long-term disease, or by the levodopa absorption being blocked by absorption of dietary protein.

Less Common Fluctuations
Many of these less common symptoms are non-motor in nature, but they are usually associated with motor fluctuations (slow spells):

- pain and numbness in the legs or arms; abdominal pain may also occur
- restless legs
- sweating
- urinary frequency
- drooling and increased difficulty swallowing
- depression, anxiety, reduced memory and hallucinations; some people also experience panic, hyperventilation (uncontrollable fast, gasping breathing), moaning and screaming while in an "off" period
- shortness of breath

One person may have a number of these symptoms. It is important that family and caregivers recognize them. Treatment to reduce motor fluctuations may improve the symptoms.

Managing Levodopa-Related Daily Mobility Fluctuations
These various fluctuations may be managed by your doctor using the following strategies:

- Add a dopamine agonist and decrease the levodopa if dyskinesias increase.
- Use a slow-release levodopa/carbidopa preparation.
- Supplement the slow-release levodopa/carbidopa with regular levodopa/carbidopa.
- Add a COMT inhibitor (see below).
- Use more frequent, smaller doses of levodopa (often without increasing the daily dosage).
- Chew or break tablets of regular levodopa/carbidopa so the drugs start taking effect sooner.
- Take chewed tablets of regular levodopa/carbidopa with a carbonated beverage, which may further speed the onset of action.
- Try liquid levodopa (see below).
- Observe the impact of high-protein meals on the levodopa effect; altering the relative timing of levodopa and food may improve the duration of the drug's effect.
- Consider a surgical procedure.

Other ways to enhance the effectiveness of levodopa include:
- inserting a tube through the wall of the abdomen and into the small bowel to allow direct delivery of nutrients and levodopa; this also improves nutrition if swallowing is poor
- preparing levodopa in a liquid form and drinking it every hour or two (this is only done under careful supervision; most people find it very cumbersome)

Dyskinesias

These involuntary movements of the face, arms, legs or trunk should not be confused with tremor. Tremor is more smooth and rhythmic, whereas dyskinesias tend to be jerky (*chorea*) and twisting (*dystonia*). Dyskinesias are often more prominent in people with more advanced disease, and are worse on the more affected side. Family may first observe these movements as restlessness (especially in the legs) or an inability to sit still.

Dyskinesias caused by levodopa treatment occur in up to 80 percent of people who have had Parkinson's for more than fifteen years. They frequently accompany mobility fluctuations such as "wearing off" and "on-off" effects, and they are worsened by stress or activity. They are thought to be caused by pulsatile stimulation (see "The Levodopa Debate," above). They will decrease if the dose is reduced, but then the parkinsonism may be worse. Dopamine agonists cause fewer episodes of dyskinesia than levodopa, and the probability of developing dyskinesias is lower in people who are only on dopamine agonist therapy. For a while it was hoped that early use of antioxidants such as vitamin E or selegiline might protect against the onset of dyskinesias and motor fluctuations; unfortunately, this has not proved to be true.

There are various patterns of dyskinesia:

Peak-dose dyskinesia: this earliest, most common form occurs at the peak of levodopa's effect, and people tend to have maximum involuntary movements when they are most active. In the early stages the dyskinesias are usually well tolerated and are easy to control by reducing the doses of levodopa. However, as the disease advances this reduction in levodopa is no longer tolerable, and other strategies must be tried (see below).

Diphasic dyskinesia (onset and end-of-dose dyskinesia) occurs shortly after taking levodopa, when the antiparkinsonian effect commences, and also when the effect of the drug is wearing off. Onset dyskinesias are thus followed by an "on" period, while end-of-dose dyskinesias are followed by an "off" period. Ten to fifteen percent of people with Parkinson's develop diphasic dyskinesia, but some have only the onset or only the end-of-dose phase. Severe leg kicking is often part of the pattern. Controlled-release levodopa/carbidopa is not recommended for this problem, as it will prolong the duration of the dyskinesias.

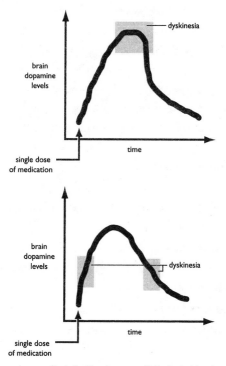

Peak dyskinesia versus diphasic dyskinesia

Dystonias are involuntary movements involving more continuous muscular contractions. Dystonia may be diphasic, peak or end-of-dose. It is more sustained when the levodopa effect is wearing off, and more intermittent and brief at the peak of the drug's effect. (It can also occur in people who are not yet on levodopa, but this is less common.) Dystonia usually involves the head and neck, with the head turning, the face contracting, the eyes blinking or the tongue thrusting outwards.

Early-morning and end-of-dose (off-period) dystonias usually affect the feet or legs, and are characterized by painful muscle contractions similar to cramps. They are related to low dopamine levels and are on the side most affected by parkinsonism.

To relieve early-morning foot dystonic movements, your doctor can try:

- a slow-release preparation of levodopa taken the night before
- a dopamine agonist taken the night before
- a dose of levodopa on wakening
- lithium (normally used as a mood stabilizer)
- botulinum toxin injections (to weaken and relax the muscles that are overactive)

To relieve "peak" dystonic movements, the following can be tried:

- a lower dose of levodopa
- adding (or increasing) a dopamine agonist and decreasing the levodopa
- botulinum toxin injections
- a surgical procedure (see "Surgical Procedures," below)

For tips on relieving "end-of-dose" dystonic movements, see the treatment suggestions for daily mobility fluctuations.

Akathisia occurs in one-quarter of Parkinson's patients, and in patients with fluctuations, and it can appear in either the "on" or the "off" phase. It is seen as restlessness or an inability to sit or lie still, and is associated with a conscious urge to move. This is different from dyskinesias, in which people may not be aware of their movements.

Akathisia can happen before levodopa treatment begins, but usually starts once the person is on levodopa. It may be a serious problem at night, causing insomnia. Minor sedatives (such as clonazepam or a dopamine agonist) may help, if adjusting the dose of levodopa does not resolve the problem. To relieve dyskinesias, your doctor may:

- reduce the daily intake of levodopa, or use more frequent, smaller doses
- add amantadine
- combine a dopamine agonist with a reduced dose of levodopa
- reduce or stop the use of selegiline
- reduce or stop anticholinergics, and observe the possible effect of other drugs with anticholinergic effects, such as antidepressants and bladder drugs
- add clozapine (a special type of dopamine-blocking medication)
- consider a surgical procedure

Dopamine Agonists

Dopamine agonists are a class of medications that are not converted to dopamine in the brain, as levodopa is. Instead, they bind directly to the dopamine receptors on the walls of brain cells, like a key fitting into a lock. By directly stimulating the dopamine receptors, they mimic some of the effects of dopamine in the brain.

We now know that there are at least five subtypes of dopamine receptors; in other words, the dopamine "key" fits into five different "locks." Drugs are being developed that selectively fit just one or two locks.

There are currently four different oral dopamine agonists available to treat Parkinson's disease in the U.S. and Canada: two "old" ones, bromocriptine and pergolide, and two "new" ones, ropinirole and pramipexole. All have been shown to be effective and all can be used in place of levodopa in the early stages of the disease, but most patients will eventually need levodopa.

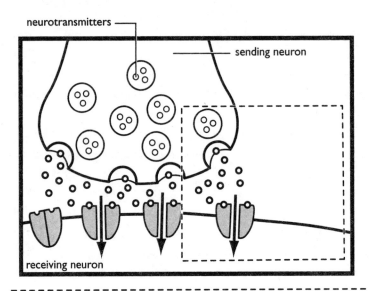

neurotransmitters

sending neuron

receiving neuron

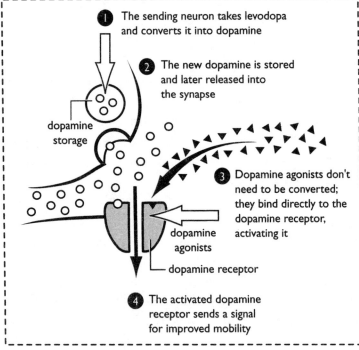

1. The sending neuron takes levodopa and converts it into dopamine

2. The new dopamine is stored and later released into the synapse

dopamine storage

3. Dopamine agonists don't need to be converted; they bind directly to the dopamine receptor, activating it

dopamine agonists

dopamine receptor

4. The activated dopamine receptor sends a signal for improved mobility

Dopamine transmission

In later stages of Parkinson's, dopamine agonists can improve motor fluctuations and reduce "off" times, and they are less likely to cause dyskinesias than levodopa. Very few studies have compared dopamine agonists against each other. There is a suggestion that the newer agonists may be more potent than bromocriptine in improving symptoms, but this has not yet been proven. The newer dopamine agonists are also being investigated to see if they can slow the progression of the disease.

What Are the Drawbacks of Dopamine Agonists?
Dopamine agonists are more expensive than levodopa. They are less potent—especially in later stages of the disease—and more complex to use, usually take longer to reach effective doses and have more side effects. However, because they tend to cause fewer dyskinesias and motor fluctuations, they are being used increasingly on their own in the early stages of the disease, especially in younger people.

The most frequent adverse side effects are nausea and vomiting, lightheadedness on standing (postural hypotension), drowsiness, constipation and psychiatric reactions (hallucinations and confusion). The nausea and postural hypotension tend to occur when treatment begins, and to diminish over days to weeks as tolerance develops. Because of the possible psychiatric reactions, dopamine agonists have to be prescribed with caution for older people, or people with preexisting psychiatric illness.

A very rare side effect, called sudden onset of sleep, or sleep attacks, has been reported in some people taking dopamine agonists; they fall asleep abruptly, without any warning. This can obviously be very serious—if, for example, they are driving at the time. It should be reported to the doctor immediately, so that the medication can be adjusted appropriately. (These spells have also been reported in people taking only levodopa, but they seem to happen less often with levodopa than with the dopamine agonists.)

Certain serious but infrequent side effects are associated with the older dopamine agonists (bromocriptine and pergolide) but are unlikely with the newer ones (pramipexole and ropinirole). These include lung and abdominal wall thickening (fibrosis) and erythromelalgia (a painful reddish skin discoloration over the legs).

How Are Dopamine Agonists Taken?

Because these drugs are complicated to use, therapy should be started under the supervision of an experienced neurologist. The basic principles are to:

- start them at a very low dosage
- increase the dose slowly
- (in many cases) reduce the levodopa at the same time

It is important to understand that the agonists rarely relieve symptoms at the lowest dose levels; don't become discouraged or discontinue the therapy. It may take several weeks of gradually increasing the dose before you notice the benefits. Also, these medications should not be stopped suddenly; doing so can make symptoms significantly worse, and can even result in a life-threatening medical emergency called neuroleptic malignant syndrome.

Neuroleptic malignant syndrome

In neuroleptic malignant syndrome, people become extremely stiff, confused and drowsy, and develop a high fever. This is thought to happen because of a sudden drop in the dopamine level in the brain. Treatment is aimed at restoring the dopamine level and controlling the fever.

COMT Inhibitors

COMT (catechol-O-methyl transferase) is an enzyme found in both the brain and the peripheral nervous system (which extends throughout the body). COMT helps break down levodopa; therefore, if its action can be inhibited (reduced), more levodopa will remain available to the brain and the rest of the nervous system. Both entacapone and tolcapone inhibit the action of COMT in the peripheral nervous system, and tolcapone also has a mild inhibiting effect within the brain itself. COMT inhibitors have no effect except when used in conjunction with levodopa. A new medication that combines entacapone, levodopa and carbidopa in a single tablet has just become available in the United States.

What Are the Benefits and Drawbacks of COMT Inhibitors?

Many studies have shown that these drugs do prolong the availability of levodopa, and improve the response to it. They are used mostly for people who are having difficulty with motor fluctuations (e.g., end-of-dose or wearing-off effect), but they have also been shown to benefit people without fluctuations.

Since COMT inhibitors keep more levodopa available to the brain, they are associated with increased levodopa side effects—dyskinesia and, less often, confusion and/or hallucinations. Because of this, the dose of levodopa may have to be reduced by up to 30 percent. For people who already have a moderate amount of dyskinesia, the total daily levodopa dose may have to be decreased by 20 percent to 30 percent right at the time the COMT inhibitor is started.

In addition to dyskinesias, hallucinations and confusion, the most common side effects of COMT inhibitors are nausea, diarrhea and urine discoloration (dark orange or red).

Tolcapone was the first of the COMT inhibitors to be approved. One of the uncommon side effects of tolcapone (but not entacapone)—affecting 1 to 3 percent of patients—is an elevation of liver enzymes. If this effect is detected early, it can be reversed by stopping the medication. Unfortunately, three people died as a result of sudden liver failure because the elevated enzymes were not detected in time. This resulted in the medication being withdrawn from use in many countries. It is still available in the United States, and on a very restricted basis in Canada, but anyone taking it has to have frequent liver function tests.

In general, however, COMT inhibitors have few side effects and are easy to administer. Because they have a rapid onset of action, if side effects like dyskinesia are going to develop, they are normally seen within the first twenty-four to forty-eight hours. It is therefore a good idea to start these drugs early in the week; if trouble does arise, it may be easier to contact your physician.

Monoamine Oxidase-B Inhibitors

Monoamine oxidase-B is an enzyme that inactivates dopamine in the brain; if the action of the enzyme is inhibited, more dopamine will be available to the brain. Selegiline, a drug that inhibits monoamine oxidase-B, may be used alone to give some relief of symptoms in newly diagnosed, very mildly affected patients, and may delay the need for levodopa for up to one year. However, for most people it has only a small effect on Parkinson's symptoms. When someone who is already on levodopa goes onto selegiline as well, a 10 percent to 30 percent reduction in the levodopa may be required. Despite early hopes that selegiline would delay the progression of Parkinson's, studies to date have shown minimal, if any, protective effect.

What Are the Drawbacks of Selegiline?

Selegiline also causes a number of uncommon but serious side effects; these are more common in people who are also on lev-

---

Interactions between selegiline and other drugs

Selegiline should not be used with the painkiller meperidine. It should not be used with cold and sinus remedies containing ephedrine; the combination may raise blood pressure. Caution is recommended when selegiline is taken with any antidepressant (such as a tricyclic antidepressant or a serotonin reuptake inhibitor), as there is a potential interaction between antidepressants and selegiline, but this interaction is very rare. However, selegiline should be discontinued about ten days before any major surgery, if possible, because it could interact with anesthetics used during the operation.

---

odopa. Confusion, hallucinations, increased dyskinesias and lowering of blood pressure (postural hypotension) are the most frequent. Special care must be used when older people are on selegiline, and the drug should not be used by anyone with a history of confusion or hallucinations. Other common side effects include heartburn and/or nausea, insomnia, dizziness and dry mouth.

Selegiline is a very long-lasting drug, and the chemical changes it causes in the brain may persist for six to eight weeks after the drug is stopped. Although the usual dose is 5 mg twice daily, much smaller doses can be effective. People who have side effects from higher doses may benefit, with no side effects, from doses as low as half a tablet (2.5 mg) once a day, or even one to three times per week. Overall, this medication is normally well tolerated, but since it may cause insomnia it is better taken early in the day.

Amantadine

Amantadine was first developed as an antiviral agent, and by chance was discovered to have antiparkinsonian effects. It provides mild to modest improvement—alleviating tremor, rigidity and bradykinesia, and perhaps smoothing out the wearing-off effect.

Amantadine's exact mechanism is unclear. It may act by enhancing the release of dopamine, or by blocking the reuptake (reabsorption) of dopamine. Recent studies suggest that amantadine may block the action of another chemical messenger, glutamate, and that blocking this may account for some of its anti-parkinsonian efficacy. It has also been suggested that amantadine improves survival in Parkinson's patients, possibly by its glutamate-blocking mechanism, but this is far from proven. However, it has been shown that amantadine does improve levodopa-induced dyskinesias in the later stages of the disease, and that this effect can last more than two years.

What Are the Drawbacks of Amantadine?
Amantadine is easy to use and normally well tolerated. Among its uncommon side effects are confusion, leg swelling, nausea, blurred vision, dry mouth, red mottled skin color on the legs, and insomnia. Amantadine should not be used by people with cognitive deficits, as it can increase their confusion and further impair their memory. It is generally discontinued for people having difficulty with confusion and/or hallucinations. However, in rare instances the withdrawal of amantadine increases confusion and agitation, and the drug has to be restarted.

Amantadine is excreted by the kidneys, so it is used in lower doses and with more caution for anyone with kidney dysfunction. If leg swelling is a problem, it may help to take the drug on alternate days. If amantadine is going to be stopped it should be withdrawn slowly; it has been suggested that sudden withdrawal may possibly cause neuroleptic malignant syndrome.

Anticholinergics
When the brain's level of dopamine is depleted by Parkinson's disease, this upsets the balance between dopamine and a chemical messenger called acetylcholine. Anticholinergics block the

action of acetylcholine, and this improves the balance between acetylcholine and dopamine.

Anticholinergic drugs have been used in the treatment of Parkinson's disease for decades, since before levodopa therapy was available. Their major effect is on parkinsonian tremor; they have little or no effect on slowness or stiffness. Since all the anticholinergics are similar in action, there are few reasons for trying more than one of them. The most commonly used are trihexyphenidyl and benztropine.

What Are the Drawbacks of Anticholinergics?

Although anticholinergics are sometimes used for younger people who are troubled mainly by tremor, side effects are common; these drugs are now being used much less than in the past. They tend to slow memory and cause confusion. They may aggravate dyskinesias. Other common side effects include blurred vision, dry mouth, constipation, hallucinations, urinary retention, impotence, rapid heartbeat, and nausea and vomiting. Older people should not take anticholinergics, as they may trigger glaucoma.

If anticholinergics are used, they should be started and stopped very gradually—over many weeks or months. Sudden withdrawal may markedly aggravate parkinsonism, whereas very slow, cautious withdrawal may hardly be noticed. However, most experienced Parkinson neurologists now seldom prescribe these drugs.

General Tips for Taking Medication

- Use a pillbox (dosette) with separate compartments to store medications for a day, especially if you are going out. This helps you organize the individual doses, and lets you avoid carrying bottles. Prepare the day's drugs the night before, or in the morning.

- Use a pill timer if you are taking frequent doses of medication; the timer sounds an alarm when each set of medications should be taken. Many different types are available; ask your doctor or pharmacist.
- Use a pill cutter, available at any drugstore, to split pills for half-tablet or quarter-tablet doses. A nail clipper with a straight cutting edge also works.
- Keep medication at your bedside at night, especially if you are slow in the morning.
- Carry extra medication when going out, in case the trip takes longer than you anticipate. Take a day's supply of drugs.
- In case of emergency, carry a list of all your medications and dosages and the times these should be taken.
- If you are having vision or hand problems, ask your pharmacist for large-print labels or non-childproof containers.
- Understand as much as you can about your medications.
- Use one pharmacy for all your drugs, including those that have nothing to do with Parkinson's. Get to know the pharmacist, and discuss your drugs and possible interactions between them.
- To swallow medications more easily, first take a sip of water to wet your mouth. Dip the tablets or capsules into water before placing them in your mouth. Follow them with a full glass of water.
- If swallowing pills is a significant problem, try chewing a banana or adding the pills to warm applesauce or some other pureed fruit. This allows the pills to slide down more easily.
- If confusion or hallucinations occur, all drugs for all conditions should be suspected and reviewed by your doctor.

Drug Therapy for Side Effects

Remember that medication for Parkinson's is very much tailored to the individual. You may have frequent changes in the dosages and timing of your drugs, and your treatment plan may be very different from someone else's. Improvement in mobility must often be weighed against the side effects of the drugs, and many people tolerate bothersome dyskinesias for the sake of improved mobility. Other side effects, such as hallucinations, may be so bothersome that both patients and their families prefer to decrease the levodopa and other drugs to avoid them, even if this means losing some mobility.

Hallucinations

As medication increases, hallucinations are likely to increase as well. Unfortunately, many of the drugs normally used to control hallucinations will make the Parkinson's worse. Clozapine may be helpful, but it causes drowsiness and sometimes has more serious side effects, so careful monitoring is necessary. Olanzapine or risperidone is sometimes used, especially for someone who is on levodopa only, but they too cause drowsiness and have other side effects, so they are not a first choice. A newer drug, quetiapine, has been giving excellent results in suppressing hallucinations and delirium, and has become the preferred drug for these problems. If the hallucinations cannot be controlled through medication, it may be necessary to reduce the drug that is causing them.

Confusion

As noted earlier, many drugs used to treat Parkinson's can cause confusion. On top of this, almost any drug—pain medication, tranquilizers, antidepressants, even drugs to reduce stomach acid—can make a confused person more confused.

Confusion and hallucinations

Drugs that may cause confusion and hallucinations include:

- levodopa
- dopamine agonists
- anticholinergics
- selegiline
- amantadine

Donepezil, rivastigmine or galantamine, drugs used to treat memory loss, may be helpful. If not, the confusion may have to be accepted for the sake of the medication's benefits.

Surgical Procedures

Surgical treatment of Parkinson's disease is not new; operations have been performed since the 1940s. However, with newer surgical techniques available, and with the realization that there are limits to what we can do with medication, there is now renewed interest in surgical interventions.

One of the new advances is stereotactic surgery, in which needle probes are guided to exact areas of the brain, using sophisticated computerized imaging (CT scans and magnetic resonance imaging). Stereotactic techniques are now used for lesioning procedures and for the placement of deep brain stimulators (see below). They are also used for transplant-implant surgeries, but these are still considered experimental; see Chapter 7.

Why Is Brain Surgery Used?

In learning more about the anatomy and function of the brain, we have come to recognize that certain areas of the brain are overactive in people with Parkinson's disease. Three of these areas are the thalamus, the pallidum and the subthalamic nucleus. These are currently the main targets for two surgical approaches: lesioning procedures, and the placement of deep brain stimulators. Both procedures are intended to decrease or stop the function of a particular brain area.

What Is the Surgery Like for the Patient?

The patient remains awake in the operating room while these procedures are being performed, because the surgeon needs the patient's feedback about his or her eyesight, abnormal sensations and extra movements; this information is vital because it helps the surgeon verify what is happening in which part of the brain. For some procedures, the surgeon also stimulates and/or records the activity of cells as probes are being inserted, to help confirm that the desired location has been found. (The target varies, depending on which symptoms are most disabling for this individual.) Since the procedures usually last three to six hours, they can be very demanding to the patient.

How Much Does the Surgery Help?

A successful procedure gives the person extra benefit beyond what drug therapy can supply. It can give better tremor control, decrease dyskinesia, improve painful cramping, and extend the duration of time spent in an optimum "on" time. In most cases it does not eliminate the need for medications, but it can dramatically improve the person's life. Unfortunately, surgery is not a cure, and it does not affect the natural progression of the disease.

Can Anyone with Parkinson's Have This Surgery?

Not all patients are candidates for these procedures. As there is a small risk of severe, permanent complications from stereotactic surgery, the only people considered are those who are severely disabled, are unable to cope with the activities of daily living, and require some assistance. Even then, all other medical options should be exhausted first.

Candidates need to be otherwise in good general health, cooperative, not depressed or cognitively impaired, and still responsive enough to levodopa that they can walk unsustained for at least a few hours a day. People with severe heart, lung, kidney or liver disease, or incurable cancer, are also not considered.

Lesioning Procedures
In a lesioning procedure, the surgeon uses a probe to destroy part of the brain, to diminish the excessive activity that is causing the unwanted symptoms. When the procedure is done on the thalamus it is called a thalamotomy. When it is done on the pallidum it is called a pallidotomy. (A few people have undergone stereotactic lesions of the subthalamic nucleus—called a subthalamotomy—but there is a concern that this procedure may cause extra abnormal movements, called ballism, and it is currently not being performed in most centers.) With all lesioning procedures, destruction is permanent and not reversible.

Thalamotomy
Thalamotomy is very effective in improving or completely relieving tremor in the majority of people who have the procedure. There are many different sub-regions within the thalamus, but the region currently being targeted to treat tremor is called the ventral intermediate (Vim) nucleus (also known as the ventrolateral nucleus). The lesion is made in the thalamus on the opposite side of the body from the tremor being treated, because most of the pathways connecting the rest of the body to the brain actually cross to the opposite side of the brain; in other words, the right side of the body is generally controlled by the left half of the brain. (Someone who has severe tremor of both arms may have an operation on both sides of the brain.)

Although it is effective in many people, about 15 percent of thalamotomy patients have their tremor recur, usually within three months of the procedure. Thalamotomy offers little prolonged improvement in other features of the disease, such as slowness or gait problems. Since most people with Parkinson's are not disabled by their tremor, only a minority are considered for this procedure.

Pallidotomy

More than 80 percent of the benefit of pallidotomy is in improving dyskinesia caused by levodopa. A lesion is made in an area of the pallidum called the ventroposterolateral part of the internal segment of the globus pallidus (Gpi). The majority of the improvement in dyskinesia will be on the side opposite the lesion, and this seems to be a long-lasting effect. (Some improvement will be seen on the same side as the lesion, but this is usually temporary.)

There will be a reduction in tremor, rigidity and bradykinesia, but the extent of these is more variable, and the duration of benefit shorter, than for dyskinesia. (Pallidotomy has a less consistent effect on tremor than does thalamotomy.) Pallidotomy also improves gait, freezing and postural stability, but this effect is usually lost within six months. Pain associated with abnormal muscle spasms and rigidity is often almost totally abolished.

In general, a pallidotomy can improve the level of parkinsonian symptoms the person had in "off" phases, but—except for dyskinesias—there is no improvement in the symptoms during the "on" phase. In other words, people are no better than they used to be in their best "on" phases with medication, but those "on" phases last longer. Most people remain on about the same levodopa level following pallidotomy. However, because they now have better control of their dyskinesia, some can tolerate higher doses of levodopa.

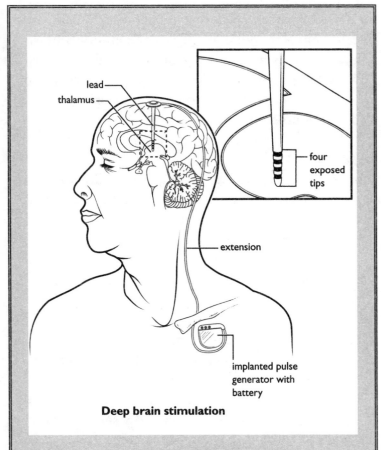

Deep brain stimulation

The "brain" of the brain probe

At the tip of the probe used for deep brain stimulation are four different contact sites that can be used to supply electrical pulses. After insertion, the probe is programmed to give a certain pattern of pulses, and it can be reprogrammed as necessary to adjust the electrical variables and/or change the contact site being used. This allows the neurologist a certain amount of flexibility in the deep brain stimulation, over the long term. Programming the stimulator can be very complex. In some cases it takes more than thirty hours, over multiple office visits, to find the optimum settings.

What Can Go Wrong?

Both thalamotomy and pallidotomy are associated with potentially serious complications. There is a 2 to 3 percent chance of having a significant stroke (bleeding into the brain tissue) during the procedure, with the risk of death less than 1 percent. Speech and swallowing difficulties occur in less than 10 percent of people who have a procedure performed on one side only, but the risk is significantly increased (up to 30 percent) when the procedure is done on both sides. Difficulties with memory and thinking can worsen—again, especially if the procedure is performed bilaterally (on both sides); for this reason, people with moderate or greater memory disturbances are not candidates for these operations. Significant weight gain has been reported in people who have had pallidotomies. Persistent difficulty with vision used to be a problem following pallidotomy; however, with improved surgical techniques this has become rare. Temporary side effects may include confusion, facial weakness or a seizure.

Deep Brain Stimulation
Deep brain stimulation (DBS) for Parkinson's disease was first tried in the late 1980s. The procedure involves inserting a permanent probe into one or more target areas of the brain. The probe is connected to a device similar to a heart pacemaker, which supplies regular high-frequency electrical pulses to those areas of the brain—not to stimulate their function, but to decrease it or stop it altogether. Like lesioning procedures, DBS can be done bilaterally (on both sides of the brain rather than just one side). Unlike lesioning, stimulation does not destroy brain tissue.

Thalamic Stimulation
Deep brain stimulation aimed at the thalamus (the Vim nucleus) has been shown to be highly effective in reducing tremor, with success rates similar to those of thalamotomy. For people with Parkinson's the effect continues for at least a few years, although for some people with essential tremor the

improvement decreases with time. If the stimulation is turned off, the tremor rapidly returns. Like thalamotomy, thalamic DBS does not improve the slowness or gait of people with Parkinson's, but it may have some effect on dyskinesias.

The risks related to speech, swallowing and memory difficulties seem to be less with bilateral stimulation than with bilateral lesioning. The risk of having a stroke during the DBS procedure is about 2 percent—similar to the risk during lesioning. It's fairly common to have temporary side effects—numbness, tingling, pulling sensations and/or double vision—while the programming is being done.

The major drawbacks of having stimulation rather than lesioning are that:

- the implanted hardware may become infected (in which case it has to be removed)
- the equipment may fail or break
- the battery has to be replaced (every three to five years for an implanted device)
- the procedure is more expensive because of the hardware

Effects of stereotactic procedures on different targets

	subthalamic nucleus stimulation	thalamic stimulation or lesion	pallidal stimulation or lesion
tremor	+++	+++	++
slowness	+++	0	+(+)
stiffness	+++	+	++
dyskinesia	++*	+	+++

+ = mildly effective
++ = moderately effective
+++ = greatly effective
0 = no effect

*when levodopa dose is reduced

Pallidal Stimulation

Not as many people have had DBS of the pallidum. Like pallidotomy, pallidal stimulation has a dramatic effect on abnormal movements induced by levodopa, but a variable effect on parkinsonian signs and symptoms; some people are greatly improved, others only mildly so. Programming the stimulators can be difficult, because some of the settings that give the best control of dyskinesias may also increase the bradykinesia, and seem to block the benefit derived from levodopa.

Subthalamic Nucleus Stimulation

The subthalamic nucleus is becoming the preferred target of DBS for people with Parkinson's. Tremor, stiffness and slowness are all clearly improved by this procedure. There can be such a marked improvement in fluctuations that some people no longer have any "off" time.

Subthalamic nucleus stimulation does not directly relieve levodopa-induced dyskinesias. However, because it does so much to improve all the major parkinsonian symptoms, the levodopa doses can be drastically reduced, so the dyskinesias abate. In rare cases the levodopa is stopped completely and the patients remain fully mobile. Speech can be improved in some people but not in others.

No well-conducted clinical trials comparing pallidal to subthalamic stimulation have been performed, but experience suggests that the subthalamic stimulation may have clinical and practical advantages, and it is the surgery of choice at most centers.

SEVEN

Hope for the Future

In research lies hope for everyone who must live with chronic illness. In particular, this is the most exciting and optimistic time in history for brain research. New knowledge, new treatment concepts and new therapies are being developed at an amazing pace, giving people with neurological disorders comfort and hope in their daily struggle.

From Understanding to Healing

Many of the latest "tools" we are using in our quest to treat brain disorders come from our growing understanding of basic cell function in other areas, such as cancer. It is becoming clear that seemingly different brain diseases often share common cell mechanisms, so what we learn about one disorder may be relevant to others as well. For example, some Alzheimer's patients develop features of parkinsonism; similarly, memory-enhancing drugs developed for Alzheimer's may help some Parkinson's patients. The illnesses are quite different, yet they apparently involve similar chemical problems. The more we learn about one brain disease, the better we may be able to deal with another.

These days, researchers are focusing their efforts on:
- understanding the factors that cause a loss of dopamine cells

- finding ways to protect the brain against Parkinson's
- diagnosing the disorder early, even before symptoms appear
- preventing the progression of the disorder
- restoring affected neurons, perhaps with growth factors (see below)
- finding new ways to deliver drug treatments
- developing new methods and materials for transplants and other surgery

Looking for New Approaches

It is now accepted that not all the problems people have from Parkinson's disease are related to the loss of dopamine cells in the substantia nigra. Defects in other chemical systems (such as the serotonin system and the noradrenergic system) play major roles in depression, and in problems of thinking and sleeping. Researchers are just beginning to explore these other chemical systems, and how they may be contributing to the disease. Many of the drug treatments now being explored are aimed in these new directions.

Here is a brief overview of some current lines of research. It's too soon to say how successful they will be. Some will probably not work out, for one reason or another; others may give us small but steady improvements in treatment. One day—sooner or later—we will find a practical, effective treatment for this disease, and the loss and heartbreak it causes.

Drug Research

Lysoganglioside

GM1 is a natural component of brain cells that was proposed to help stimulate growth factors in the brain. In animal models of Parkinson's, GM1 has been shown to help restore the function of damaged dopamine cells, and to protect against further damage. In preliminary studies in people with Parkinson's, it has likewise been shown to improve function. Unfortunately, GM1 had a number of drawbacks; it had to be injected, and the original compound, in its unpurified form, had significant side effects.

Lysoganglioside is a newer, semi-synthetic derivative of GM1 that can be given orally to laboratory animals, and shows promise as a replacement. It may give the benefits of GM1 without the side effects.

Glutamate Antagonists

Researchers believe that some late levodopa complications, including fluctuations and dyskinesias, result from excessive activity of the brain's glutamate receptors, and that this excess may cause neurons to die, and may contribute to the progression of the disease. Amantadine appears to work as a glutamate antagonist, blocking the receptors and diminishing this excessive activity. Studies in humans have suggested that it may slow the progression of the disease, but this is still far from proven. A number of other possible glutamate agonists are now being studied. One is rimantadine, a longer-acting derivative of amantadine. Others are budipine, remacemide and dextromethorphan. If this new approach to restoring neuron function proves to be successful, it may become an alternative to surgery.

Adenosine Receptor Blockers

Adenosine A_{2A} antagonists act by inhibiting the action of cells that are involved in the complex interconnections within the brain. In animal models of Parkinson's, they have been shown to help reduce motor fluctuations without worsening dyskinesia. Some monkey models have also suggested that this compound could have a protective effect on dopamine cells. A number of these inhibitors have been produced, but a compound called KW-6002 is the one farthest along in development. Early reports suggest that it is well tolerated in humans, and show improvements in motor function similar to those seen in animal models. Larger studies are nearing completion in people with later-stage Parkinson's. If they are positive, this will provide a much-needed new class of treatment options for such individuals.

Nicotine Receptor Enhancers

Since smoking seems to decrease the risk of developing of Parkinson's, there has been great interest in studying nicotine receptors. Nicotine is presumed to be responsible for the effect, yet the use of nicotine patches has not been shown to be helpful. Now, highly selective compounds have been developed that bind to specific subtypes of nicotine receptors in the brain. These compounds (such as SIB 1508Y and ABT-418) are thought to work by enhancing the amount of the neurotransmitters dopamine and acetylcholine released in the brain. Early trials of these compounds suggest that they may help, not only with the motor impairments of Parkinson's, but also with memory.

New Methods of Delivery

Trials have been done on new ways of administering drugs. Apomorphine (a dopamine agonist) is currently administered by injections; by continuous infusion under the skin; by a skin patch similar to the transdermal patches commonly used to deliver certain hormones or to wean smokers off nicotine; or sublingually (placed under the tongue, and absorbed through the thin tissue there. The sublingual approach is effective, but is limited by the fact that apomorphine use is associated with significant nausea and irritation of the mouth). Another dopamine agonist, rotigotine, has been developed to be absorbed through the skin. Studies of this drug in transdermal patches are in the final phases, and it's expected that transdermal rotigotine will be on the market within the next few years.

For some people with Parkinson's, the benefits of levodopa are limited by slow stomach emptying and poor drug absorption. Levodopa ethylester is a highly soluble oral solution that may help these people combat disabling fluctuations and dyskinesias that are not controlled by regular or slow-release levodopa/carbidopa.

Gene Therapy

Exactly what is gene therapy? There are many different definitions. The simplest is that gene therapy is treatment of a disease by genetic manipulation. Hundreds of diseases are being targeted with various types of gene therapy, and the list now includes Parkinson's.

Early gene therapy was aimed at very rare genetic diseases involving a problem with a single gene; the goal was to fix that one gene defect. As Parkinson's is rarely due to a single gene defect, this strategy will not work. Instead, the goal is to target any number of pathways, and try to genetically modify what that pathway is doing. Many different approaches have been suggested. For example, you could try to insert genes into the brain that control dopamine cell survival, or enhance dopamine production.

Inhibitory Factors

One very ingenious technique that is currently being performed in a clinical trial uses a natural inhibitory factor found in the brain, glutamic acid decarboxylase (GAD). The GAD factor is inserted into a virus that can carry it into brain cells. Some people in this clinical trial are getting regular deep brain stimulation of the subthalamic nucleus, which is overactive in people with Parkinson's. Others are getting DBS as well as an injection of the virus with the GAD factor attached, to inhibit the firing of the subthalamic nucleus. The results of this trial are being closely followed, to see if this type of treatment is not only effective but also safe.

Growth Factors

Growth factors are compounds found throughout the body that enhance the function, replication or survival of targeted cells. We have known for more than a decade that certain factors enhance the survival and function of brain cells. Glial-derived neurotrophic factor (GDNF) is one of the most potent and best studied of these, and it has been shown to have a beneficial effect on dopamine cells in experimental models of Parkinson's. The problem is that GDNF is a large compound that doesn't cross from the blood into the brain. Early attempts were made to inject it into the fluid-filled cavities deep inside the brain, in the hope that it would diffuse into brain tissue and improve the survival and function of dopamine cells. Unfortunately, GDNF has too many side effects when it's injected this way, and it didn't diffuse as intended.

Researchers are now attempting to continuously infuse GDNF directly to the location where the dopamine cells affect the brain, via a small tube. A study of five people with advanced Parkinson's has just been reported to have had beneficial effects. The five were followed over eighteen months, and seem to have tolerated the GDNF infusions well and to have improved remarkably in motor skills and quality of life. Larger, more detailed studies are now underway in many centers to determine whether this therapy is really as effective as the initial report suggests.

Animal models have used GDNF inserted into a virus which is then injected into the animals' brains. Marked improvement is seen in the animals' function, as well as an increase in the number of dopamine-producing cells in their brains. Many technical challenges, as well as safety concerns, still need to be addressed before such treatments are used in humans. Once these challenges are met, however, it will be much less cumbersome to deliver GDNF and other growth factors into the brain through virus-based approaches.

Neuroprotection
"Neuroprotection" refers to slowing the progression of Parkinson's, and eventually finding treatments that stop the disorder from developing in the first place. Various environmental and genetic factors contribute to Parkinson's, and many different compounds have been suggested that could function as prevention or protection agents. To date, no agents have clearly been shown to affect the progress of the disease. A number of abnormal processes contribute to the progression of Parkinson's once it has started; of these, oxidative stress is the one that has been studied the longest.

The Search for Useful Antioxidants
The oxidation of dopamine is a normal chemical process that produces potentially toxic products that could damage dopamine neurons. It was hoped that selegiline, a monoamine oxidase-B inhibitor (see Chapter 6), would slow this process, but it seems not to. New drugs being tested for this purpose include transcyclopropine (which blocks both monoamine oxidase-A and monoamine oxidase-B enzymes, but is more likely to raise blood pressure), and rasagaline, a type-B inhibitor.

Coenzyme Q_{10} (CoQ_{10}) is a compound available in most health food stores. For many years it has been suggested that CoQ_{10} can protect dopamine neurons against oxidation by blocking the oxidation pathway and helping the mitochondria function. A relatively small study in humans has suggested that CoQ_{10} may slow the disease process when used in large doses (600 and 1,200 mg per day). Most health food stores carry 30 mg or 60 mg tablets, so trying to take that large a dose would be impractical, and very expensive for an as-yet-unproven therapy. However, further studies are warranted.

Although vitamin E is also an antioxidant, a large clinical study did not show it to have any effect on the progression of Parkinson's.

Combating Apoptosis

We now have compounds that can block the cell suicide (apoptosis) genes, which have been proposed as one potential mechanism of dopamine-cell death. One of these, CEP-1347, has been shown to be effective in many cell and animal models of Parkinson's. It is currently being tested on eight hundred people with Parkinson's, to see if it is well tolerated and can slow the progression of the disease. Other possible candidates for further study include creatine, N-acetyl cysteine and nicotinamide.

Stem Cells

All of us grow from tiny clusters of undifferentiated "stem" cells. Later in our development, these cells multiply and become specialized as heart cells, muscle cells, dopamine-producing brain cells and so on. Since it is theoretically possible to guide stem cells into becoming any type of cells we need, and to transplant them to where we need them, their potential in treating illnesses has generated great excitement. Researchers are just starting to identify the signals that tell a stem cell to become a brain cell. We need to do more work to understand how to coax those brain cells into becoming the specific dopamine-producing cells we want them to be. As well, there is evidence that even the adult human brain still has some capacity to grow new cells. In the future we may be able to regulate these "stem" cells that are already in the brain, and manipulate them into becoming dopamine-producing cells.

The stem-cell debate

Because human development begins with stem cells, fetal tissue—from surplus embryos created for in vitro fertilization, for example, or from umbilical cords—is the most direct source. This has led to passionate disputes over the moral issues involved, and the relative rights of human embryos versus people with serious disorders. In the United States, stem-cell research is now severely limited because of these concerns. Research continues somewhat more freely in Canada, but the issue is still hotly debated. There is hope, though, that before long fetal tissue will not be needed as the initial source for stem cells.

Tissue Implantation

Transplanting tissue into the brain as a treatment for Parkinson's has been an area of active research for many years. Since parkinsonism relates primarily to degeneration of the cells that make dopamine, the focus has been on trying to put dopamine-replacing or dopamine-enhancing cells into the basal ganglia.

Adrenal-to-Brain Implants

In the 1980s, tissue was being transplanted from one of the patient's own adrenal glands as a possible treatment for Parkinson's. Hundreds of people around the world underwent this procedure before a proper, detailed, multi-center study was done. The study showed generally poor results, without long-term benefits, and this procedure is no longer attempted.

Human Fetal Tissue Transplantation

Animal studies have shown that transplanted human fetal dopamine cells can survive and form primitive connections within the brain. Human embryonic brain cells have been transplanted into people with Parkinson's in many different countries. Early studies showed a moderate degree of benefit, and imaging studies have shown a clear increase in dopamine in the basal ganglia. Autopsies on people who received such transplants (and died for other reasons) have demonstrated that the transplanted dopamine cells can survive for many years. Despite such encouraging results, these operations are still considered experimental treatments, although they have been performed for more than twenty years in Sweden and other countries.

Two relatively large, very detailed fetal-cell studies have now been completed, involving people with advanced Parkinson's. In both these studies, placebo surgery (surgery with no actual transplant) was done for half the patients, and the other half received actual transplants. Overall, neither study showed significantly greater improvement among those who had the real transplant. Moreover, some subjects developed excessive dyskinesia that continued even after their dopamine-replacement medications were stopped.

Why did this happen when the surgery appeared effective in the earlier, non-placebo studies? Was it because of a difference in surgical techniques? Or because of the way the fetal cells were collected, or the number of fetal cells transplanted? Or were the earlier apparent benefits no more than a placebo effect? Whatever the reason, fetal-cell surgery has not been proven to improve Parkinson's, and we need further study to determine whether it will ever be an effective treatment.

Other Sources of Dopamine Tissue for Transplantation
We know that dopamine cells from pig embryos can survive and make new connections when transplanted into people with Parkinson's. Unfortunately, this surgery has not been shown to be effective in improving the recipients' overall function.

Animal studies suggest that cells from a patient's own carotid bodies may be useful "donor cells" for injection into the basal ganglia. Carotid bodies are structures on either side of the neck; they help determine our breathing rate by sensing the oxygen level in our blood. Carotid-body cells can produce many times more dopamine than fetal cells can, and they survive much better. Certain cells in the eye also produce dopamine, and these too are being explored as a possible source for transplantation.

How Do We Make More Progress?

The mass of our new understanding about Parkinson's is the result of a number of factors:

- the coordinated efforts of researchers attempting to understand brain control and function
- today's information technology, which allows an unprecedented degree of real-time scientific collaboration across great distances
- government financial support, which is essential for medical research on the scale necessary to solve the riddles of Parkinson's disease. Public funding makes good economic sense, given the immense costs of caring for people disabled by Parkinson's
- the pharmaceutical industry, which has invested many millions of dollars in developing potential therapies for people with Parkinson's, and in shepherding the more promising ones through the slow, painstaking sequence of trials and approvals

How Can You Help?

Private individuals can also play an important part in beating Parkinson's, one way or another.

Participating in Clinical Trials

Drug trials require volunteers—people who will accept treatment with a therapy whose benefits are not yet proven, people who will find time for the evaluations needed to determine which drugs work and which ones don't. All clinical studies are reviewed and approved in advance by an ethics committee (including lay representatives). Risks, benefits and the details of what is involved must be fully explained to participants before the trial begins. New therapies may be tested against established ones, or against a placebo (a simulated treatment).

While it may not seem fair that some people in a trial are not actually receiving therapy, this is the only way to be sure the new treatment is truly effective. A "placebo effect"— improved functioning without real therapy—is common among people with Parkinson's. Perhaps the hope of trying something new makes the person feel better. As well, trials often involve extra visits, tests and personal contact with medical staff; perhaps these improve the person's sense of well-being. However, studies have shown a measurable increase in brain dopamine levels in people with Parkinson's who were receiving a placebo, and some placebo benefits can last for more than six months. By testing the new therapy against a placebo, researchers can establish its true benefits, without being misled by any temporary placebo effect.

Contributing Time and Talent

Private citizens can also do major work in fund-raising, whether it's for essential research, or for the day-to-day facilities needed by people with Parkinson's and their families.

Perhaps you have personal or professional skills you can offer: supplying music, designing a website, making muffins for the bake sale. Remember, everyone's time is precious. Simply visiting a home or taking someone for an outing, giving a caregiver some free time to relax, is a contribution that will be deeply appreciated. Talk to your local Parkinson's association about what's needed, and how you can help.

Brain Donation

If you have Parkinson's, and you leave instructions that your brain can be studied after your death, you make a lasting contribution to our struggle to better understand the brain changes that take place in the course of this devastating disease. In better understanding lies our hope for more precise therapies to improve the treatment of Parkinson's, and to prevent its onset. Indeed, the original finding of brain dopamine that led to the development of levodopa therapy was made through chemical analysis of donated brain tissue.

Brain tissue banks cooperate in making tissue available to research groups worldwide. Pathologists and funeral directors are very respectful of family wishes and timelines, and there should not be any significant additional costs. If you decide to make this priceless bequest, your treatment team should be aware of your wishes. Your physician and your local Parkinson's society can help.

Yes, it's a long road to a cure for Parkinson's—but we have traveled much of it already. Every year we have better diagnosis, more effective drug therapies, more innovative surgical approaches.

We're getting closer all the time.

Table of Drug Names

Generic name	Some common drug names	Type
Anti-Parkinson drugs		
amantadine	Symmetrel, Endantadine	

levodopa
levodopa/benserazide†
levodopa/benserazide
  extended release**
levodopa/carbidopa
levodopa/carbidopa
  extended release
	Sinemet
	Prolopa, Madopar
	Madopar HBS
	
	Sinemet, Atamet
	Sinemet CR
		(see note below)

bromocriptine pergolide pramipexole ropinirole	Parlodel Permax Mirapex Requip	dopamine agonists
entacapone tolcapone	Comtan, Comtess Tasmar	COMT inhibitors
entacapone/ levodopa/carbidopa*	Stalevo	combination
selegiline	Deprenyl, Eldepryl, Carbex, Atapryl	MAOB inhibitor
benztropine ethopropazine orphenadrine procyclidine trihexyphenidyl	Cogentin Parsitan, Parsidol Disipal Kemadrin Artane	anticholinergics
For memory loss		
donepezil galantamine rivastigmine	Aricept Reminyl Excelon	cholinesterase inhibitors
For confusion		
clozapine olanzapine quetiapine risperidone	Clozaril Zyprexa Seroquel Risperdal	antipsychotics, dopamine- blocking agents
For depression		
fluoxetine paroxetine sertraline	Prozac Paxil Zoloft	selective serotonin reuptake inhibitors
amitriptyline desipramine	Elavil Norpramin	tricyclics
For anxiety and insomnia		
alprazolam clonazepam lorazepam temazepam	Xanax Klonopin, Rivotril Ativan Restoril	
For erectile dysfunction		
sildenafil tadalafil vardenafil*	Viagra Cialis Levitra	

For combinations of levodopa and carbidopa, the larger number shows the amount of levodopa and the smaller shows the amount of carbidopa. A combination of 100 mg levodopa and 25 mg carbidopa is called Sinemet 25/100 in the U.S., and Sinemet 100/25 in Canada.

*Available in U.S. only

†Available in Canada only

**Not available in North America

Generic name	Some common drug names	Type
For osteoporosis		
alendronate etidronate ibandronate* risedronate	Fosamax Didrocal Boniva Actonel	bisphosphonates
raloxifene	Evista	selective estrogen- receptor modulator
calcitonin teriparatide*	Miacalcin Forteo	hormones
For gastric emptying		
domperidone†	Motilium	
For bladder problems		
imipramine oxybutynin tolterodine	Tofranil Ditropan Detrol	

*Available in U.S. only
†Available in Canada only

Glossary

Akinesia: inability to move.

Anticholinergics: drugs that block the action of acetylcholine, a neurotransmitter in the brain.

Aphasia: a problem with any aspect of language such as reading, writing, speaking, comprehension or naming objects.

Apoptosis: a mechanism of cell death; the cell's genes "switch on" and tell it to "commit suicide."

Atypical parkinsonism: a group of conditions, resulting from the death of brain cells, that cause slowness and stiffness and sometimes tremor, but are not Parkinson's disease itself. (Also known as Parkinson-plus.)

Bradykinesia: slowness of movement, and loss of spontaneous and voluntary movement.

Carbidopa: a drug that inhibits the body from breaking down levodopa before it enters the brain. Carbidopa greatly decreases such side effects of levodopa as nausea and lightheadedness.

Classical Parkinson's: a disease caused by the death of dopamine-producing cells in a specific region of the brain (the substantia nigra) that results in stiffness, slowness and tremor. (Also known as idiopathic Parkinson's.)

Computerized tomography (CT) scan: a type of X-ray that shows "slices" of the brain or body in two dimensions.

COMT inhibitors: medications that reduce the action of COMT (catechol-O-methyl transferase), an enzyme that helps break down levodopa.

CT scan: *See* **Computerized tomography scan.**

Deep brain stimulation (DBS): a technique that uses electrical current to prevent a structure deep in the brain from functioning. The current comes from an electrode inserted in the brain and connected to a programmable power source.

Dopamine: a neurotransmitter in the brain that helps control movement and thinking.

Dopamine agonists: drugs that bind to dopamine receptors to enhance their function.

Dyskinesia: abnormal involuntary movement.

Dysphagia: difficulty with swallowing.

Dystonia: abnormal, involuntary movement causing a sustained, often twisting posture of the affected body part.

Essential tremor: a condition causing a tremor that occurs mainly when someone performs an action such as writing or drinking from a cup.

Gait disorder: any condition that causes problems with walking.

Idiopathic Parkinson's, *See* **Classical Parkinson's.**

Kinetic tremor: rhythmic movement that occurs when the person moves the affected body part, or holds it in a certain posture.

Levodopa (L-dopa): a chemical produced by the brain as one of the steps toward making dopamine. Levodopa remains the best medication for the stiffness and slowness of Parkinson's.

Lewy bodies: abnormal structures found in the brain cells of people with Parkinson's.

Magnetic resonance imaging (MRI): a technique that uses a powerful magnetic field to create very detailed pictures. Unlike CT scans, MRI scans do not involve X-rays, but give better detail.

MRI, *See* **Magnetic resonance imaging.**

Neuron: a cell in the nervous system that receives and transmits information.

Pallidotomy: an operation in which part of the brain (the pallidum) that is overactive in Parkinson's is destroyed.

Parkinson-plus, *See* **Atypical parkinsonism**

PET, *See* **Positron emission tomography.**

Positron emission tomography (PET): an imaging technique measuring functional aspects of the brain. For Parkinson's, dopamine activity can be measured and imaged.

Pulsatile stimulation: intermittent stimulation of the brain's dopamine receptors by dopamine-replacement medications.

Resting tremor: tremor when the affected body part is not being used; a typical tremor of Parkinson's.

Rigidity: abnormal increased stiffness in a body part.

Single photon emission computed tomography (SPECT): an imaging technique similar to a PET scan; it gives less detailed pictures but is easier to use and much less expensive.

SPECT, *See* **Single photon emission computed tomography.**

Stereotactic surgery: brain surgery guided by images from a CT or MRI scan.

Tardive dyskinesia: abnormal involuntary movements caused by medications that block dopamine functioning in the brain.

Thalamotomy: an operation in which part of the brain (the thalamus) is destroyed; used to improve tremor in someone with Parkinson's.

Further Resources

Organizations

U.S.A.

American Parkinson Disease
  Association, Inc.
1250 Hylan Blvd., Suite 4B
Staten Island, NY 10305
1-888-400-2732
www.apdaparkinson.com

Michael J. Fox Foundation for
  Parkinson's Research
Grand Central Station
P.O. Box 4777
New York, NY 10163
www.michaeljfox.org

National Parkinson Foundation,
  Inc.
Bob Hope Parkinson Research
  Center
1501 NW 9th Avenue
Bob Hope Road
Miami, FL 33136-1494
305-547-6666
Fax: 305-243-5595
Toll-free: 1-800-327-4545

Parkinson's Disease Foundation
710 West 168th Street
New York, NY 10032-9982
212-923-4700
Toll-free (U.S. only):
1-800-457-6676
www.pdf.org

Worldwide Education and
  Awareness for Movement
  Disorders (WE MOVE)
204 West 84th Street
New York, NY 10024
Toll-free (for materials):
  1-800-437-6682
E-mail: wemove@wemove.org
www.wemove.org

Canada

Parkinson Society Canada
4211 Yonge Street, Suite 316
Toronto, ON M2P 2A9
416-227-9700
Fax: 416-227-9600
Toll-free: 1-800-565-3000
www.parkinson.ca

Other Websites

Canadian Movement Disorder Group
www.cmdg.org

Canadian Transportation Agency
 (Accessible Transportation)
www.cta.otc.gc.ca

People Living with Parkinson's
www.plwp.org

World Parkinson Disease Association
www.wpda.org

Books

Calne, Susan, Kerry Baisley, Paula Coughlan, Trevor Hurwitz, Carole Shaw and Karol Traviss. *Taking Charge: A Guide to Living with Parkinson's*. Toronto, ON: Parkinson Society Canada, 2003.

Canadian Transport Agency. *Taking Charge of the Air Travel Experience* (brochure). Ottawa, ON: Government of Canada, 1998.

Duvoisin, Roger C., and Jacob I. Sage. *Parkinson's Disease: A Guide for Patient and Family*. Fourth edition. Philadelphia, PA: Lippincott Raven, 1996.

"Fly Smart" (brochure). Ottawa, ON: Minister of Public Works and Government Services, 2003. To order call toll-free, 1-888-222-2592, or fax 1-819-953-5686.

Fox, Michael J. *Lucky Man—A Memoir.* Winnipeg, MB: Hyperion, 2002.

Harshaw, Bill. *My Second Life: Living with Parkinson's Disease.* Toronto, ON: Dundurn, 2001.

Hauser, Robert A., Kelly E. Lyons, Rajesh Pahwa, Theresa A. Zesiewicz and Lawrence I. Golbe. *Parkinson's Disease: Questions and Answers.* Fourth edition. Cold Springs, FL: Merit, 2003.

Hutton, J. Thomas, *et al. Caring for the Parkinson Patient: A Practical Guide.* New York, NY: Prometheus, 1999.

Jahanshahi, Marjan, and C. David Marsden. *Parkinson's Disease: A Self-Help Guide.* New York: Demos, 2000.

Lieberman, Dr. Abraham. *Shaking Up Parkinson Disease.* Sudbury, MA: Jones & Bartlett, 2001.

Lieberman, Abraham N., MD, and Frank L. Williams. *Parkinson's Disease: A Complete Guide for Patients and Caregivers.* New York: Simon & Schuster, 1993.

Parkinson Society Canada. *A Manual for People Living with Parkinson's Disease.* Toronto, ON: 2003. To order a free copy call 1-800-565-3000, ext. 245.

Weiner, William J., Lisa M. Shulman and Anthony E. Lang. *Parkinson's Disease: A Complete Guide for Patients and Families.* Baltimore, MD: Johns Hopkins, 2001.

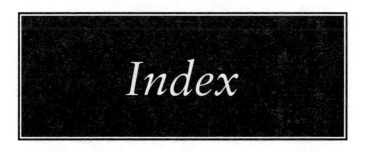

Index

Page numbers in italic indicate a figure or boxed text. For drug brands please see the table of drug names on pages 191–92.

dentures 95, 98, 103, 114
depression
    about 37, 39-40, 154
    and sexual problems 106
    and sleep problems 84
    management 81-83
desipramine 83
diarrhea 151, 163
diet and nutrition
    and bladder problems 104-5
    and blood pressure 108
    and constipation 99
    and falls 87
    and levodopa effect 155
    and sleep problems 85
    and swallowing difficulties 97-98
    and weight loss 54-55, 101-3
    calcium 47
    eating tips and devices 72, 103
    fruit spread recipe *100*
dietitians 101-2
diffuse Lewy-body disease 11-12, 38
digestive problems
    about 50
    impaired gastric emptying 52-53
    management 93-103
    nausea and vomiting 53, 150, 161,
        163, 165-67
    weight loss and poor nutrition 54-55,
        101-3
diltiazem 6
disability rating scales 31-34
diuretics 57, *104*
dizziness 165
DJ1 gene 22
docusate sodium 100
domperidone 6, 151
donepezil 170
dopamine
    deficiency of 2-3, 17-20, 82, 147
    functions 2, 17, 41, 63, 82
    production of 17
dopamine agonists
    about 29, 159-61
    adjusting 161-62
    and breastfeeding 138-39
    and pregnancy 137-38
    and sexual problems 105
    functions 77, 155, 159
    how to take 162
    side effects 29, 38, 42, 56, 109,
        161-62, *170*
dopamine-blocking drugs 134
dopamine receptors 5-7
dopamine-replacement drugs 83, 105
dressing tips and devices 70, 89
driving 140-42
drooling 50, 93, 154
drowsiness

about 41-42, 84, 161
drugs, *see also specific drugs and the
    table on pages 191-92*
    adjusting *147*
    and gait difficulties 77
    and pregnancy 136-38
    and travel 143
    causing agitation 40
    causing bladder problems 56
    causing confusion and hallucinations
        37-38, 154
    causing dry mouth 51
    causing memory problems 36, 154
    causing nausea and vomiting 53
    causing parkinsonism 3, 5-7
    causing Parkinson's 23
    causing sexual problems 57, 106
    causing sleep problems 42, 84
    causing sweating 60, 154
    causing visual or eye problems 62
    dosage 146-47
    how to take 167-68
    increasing risk of falls 87
    interactions 146-47
    medication schedule in hospital
        132-33
    research 179-81
    what to use 146-47
    when to use 145-46
dry eyes 62-63, 112-13
dry mouth 50, 93-94, 165-67
dysarthria (speech problems) 60-61,
    113-16
dyskinesia
    defined 155-56
    drug-associated 33, 45, 109, 149,
        155-57, 163, 165, 167
    management 156, 158
    types 156-58
dystonia
    body locations 43, 157-58
    defined 2, 155, 157
    in young-onset Parkinson's 2
    management 158

eating tips and devices 72, 103
elderly people *see* older people
emotional problems
    agitation 40, 83
    anxiety and panic attacks 40, 83, 154
    depression 37, 39-40, 81-84, 106, 154
employment 139-40
entacapone 163
ephedrine *165*
erythromelalgia 162
estrogen therapy
    controversies *48*
    for memory loss 116-17
    for osteoporosis 48